School Nurse Survival Guide

Note

Health and social care practice and knowledge are constantly changing and developing as new research and treatments, changes in procedures, drugs and equipment become available.

The authors, editor and publishers have, as far as is possible, taken care to confirm that the information complies with the latest standards of practice and legislation.

The School Nurse Survival Guide

edited by

Jane Wright

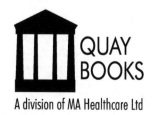

QUAY
BOOKS

A division of MA Healthcare Ltd

Quay Books Division, MA Healthcare Ltd, St Jude's Church, Dulwich Road, London
SE24 0PB

British Library Cataloguing-in-Publication Data
A catalogue record is available for this book

© MA Healthcare Limited 2012

ISBN-10: 1 85642 422 6
ISBN-13: 978 1 85642 422 7

Printed by Mimeo, Huntingdon, Cambridgeshire

Contents

Contents

Foreword

Wendy Nicholson

There are about 11.3 million school-aged children and young people in England and their health and development are vital to individuals, families and society – they are our future. The current high focus on improving the health and wellbeing of children and young people provides an opportunity for school nurses to embrace their leadership role and strengthen the delivery of public health to school-aged children and young people. The Department of Health's *Healthy Lives, Healthy People* and the *Healthy Lives, Healthy People: Update and Way Forward* reinforces the importance of health in the early and developing years.

The public health programme for children and young people – the Healthy Child Programme – is designed to offer a core, evidence-based programme of health protection, improvement and support from 5 to 19 years. The *Healthy Child Programme from 5 to 19 years old* (2009) recognises the pivotal role of the school nurse in leading and providing services and recommends staged school nursing contacts at specific milestones in a child's life.

The specialist expertise that school nurses bring to children's lives is unique. School nurses as specialist community public health practitioners are crucial to the planning, delivery and coordination of the preventative health services that children and young people need during their school-age years in order to maximise their health and wellbeing and provide strong foundations for good health and wellbeing through into adult life.

It is essential to understand the unique role and skills that the school nurse brings in terms of prevention, support and (where necessary) treatment. Due to their unique positioning within schools and local community settings, school nurses and their teams can make a positive contribution to the health and wellbeing of all school-aged children and young people. They have a crucial role in providing early help and intervention services where needed. Intervening early and working with children, young people and families to build on strengths and improve self-esteem and cohesion and, where required, referring early for more specialist help, is the most effective way of dealing with health, developmental and other issues within the family.

There is increasing knowledge about the importance of good mental health in the growing years to good outcomes in later life, and the school nursing service is holistic, seeking to address physical mental and emotional needs. Furthermore, the numbers of children and young people in mainstream education with disabilities and/or additional health needs are increasing, with much of the support falling to the school nursing services.

Getting It Right For Children, Young People And Families – Maximising the contribution of the school nursing team: Vision and Call to Action was launched by the Department of Health in 2012. The service vision and model for school offers a structured framework on which to build local services for school aged children and young people. We want a service that meets present and future needs: a service that is visible, accessible and confidential; a service which delivers universal public health and ensures that there is early help and advice available to young people at the times when they need it. School nurses need to be supported in their leadership role in the new public health system and to continue to work with children and young people ensuring they have a voice in developing services that are right for them.

This 'Survival Guide' provides comprehensive advice for existing practitioners and those new to school nursing. It offers practical and thoughtful assistance to school nurses in their work with children, young people and families. The solution-focused approaches included in this guide will assist practitioners to address challenges such as safeguarding children and the increasing number of children and young people with mental health issues. The book builds on good practice and provides an opportunity for school nurses to reflect on their practice and leadership role.

There is an opportunity for school nurses and their teams to reaffirm their role as specialist public health practitioners and to use their expertise to provide leadership to enhance the delivery of the healthy child programme, thus improving the health and wellbeing of children and young people.

Contributors

Jane Wright

MSc, Health Promotion, PG diploma, Education (Nursing), BA (Hons) Community Health Studies, Specialist Practitioner (school nursing), CPT, RGN

Jane is a Senior Lecturer and Pathway Lead for school nurses at Buckinghamshire New University. She has taught SCPHN students at the university for eight years. Before that, she worked as a community school nurse and practice teacher for nine years. Jane is on the editorial board for the *British Journal of School Nursing* and is the chairperson of the National Forum for School Health Educators. Jane was on the Department of Health steering group for the school nurse development programme in 2011.

Sharon Aldridge-Bent

MA Education, PGCert Nursing and Midwifery Education, BSc (Hons) Health Studies, District Nurse, Nurse Prescriber, RGN

Sharon is a senior lecturer at Buckinghamshire New University. She has taught on various programmes at the university for the last nine years, primarily in Community Health Care Nursing and Mentorship. Sharon has experience of project work for a strategic health authority and has also worked as a specialist nurse, Macmillan nurse and district nurse.

Kate Potter

MSc Health and Nursing Studies, PG Dip Education, BA Open, Dip HV, SRN RSCN, CPT

Kate is course leader for the SCPHN programmes at Buckinghamshire New University and Pathway Lead for health visiting. She is also course leader for the Practice Teacher Award. Prior to coming in to higher education eight years ago she worked for a considerable period of time as a health visitor and practice teacher.

Melanie Hayward
BSc SCPHN, RCN, Specialist Community Public Health Nurse, School Nursing, Buckinghamshire Healthcare NHS Trust

Melanie works as a school nurse in Buckinghamshire. She trained as a paediatric nurse at Great Ormond Street Hospital and practised in surgical and medical paediatrics as well as oncology before working as a community staff nurse for school nursing. She trained as a SCPHN in 2008–09 gaining a first class honours degree. She has a special interest in health behaviours and health promotion, specifically PSHE education.

Lynne Smith
MA, Cert Ed, BA (Hons) Public Health, CPT, RGN

Lynne qualified as a State Enrolled Nurse in 1977 at Stoke Mandeville Hospital. She has worked in a variety of nursing settings, both acute and community. She achieved a diploma in nursing in 2002 and then went on to gain a BA (Hons) in Public Health in 2004 at Reading University. Lynne works as a school nurse and obtained the certificate in teaching in 2006. She supports SCPHN students in practice. She has a dual role working with the Youth Offending Service in Bracknell developing a quality service to improve the health and wellbeing of that client group.

Rachel Cabral
BSc SCPHN, CPT, RN (child)

Rachel works as a school nurse practitioner and qualified as a practice teacher in 2011. She was a Project 2000 nurse and qualified as an RN (child) in 1993. She has worked in a variety of acute paediatric settings in the UK before coming into the community to work as a school nurse. Rachel also has experience of working abroad, teaching English to Nurse Lecturers in a school of nursing in Portugal.

Liz Torres
BSc SCPHN, RGN

Liz qualified as an adult nurse in 1994. She has had a variety of nursing jobs and came into the community in 1999 as a staff nurse in District Nursing. In 2003 she moved to school nursing as a community staff nurse and completed the SCPHN training in 2009, achieving a first class honours degree. Liz works as a school nurse practitioner and is particularly interested in developing care pathways for children with medical needs in schools. Liz is keen to share good practice and has established a group on facebook entitled 'School Nursing across the world': https://www.facebook.com/groups/175904482466056/.

Kath Lancaster

MSc Advanced Nursing Practice, BSc (Hons) Community Health Nursing, SCPHN, DIP, RN

Kath has worked in the community as both a School Nurse Practitioner and a Community Practice Teacher, directing and delivering public health information and services for young people. She has also worked as a Senior Lecturer in Specialist Public Health Nursing and as a Pathway Leader for School Nursing. More recently, Kath has been involved with the school nurse development programme at the Department of Health. Kath presently owns and directs her own Nursing Consultancy Company and has had contracts across the UK and recognition at a global level for the creation of models, frameworks and training to support public sector workforce redesign and development. Website: http://www. thelancastermodel.co.uk/.

CHAPTER 1

Working in the community as a school nurse

Jane Wright

Key themes in this chapter:

- An introduction to the content of the book
- The development of school nursing practice
- How can building partnerships promote positive health and wellbeing?
- What risks should school nurses be aware of in the community?
- What are the professional responsibilities of the school nurse?
- Delivering the Healthy Child Programme (HCP) for 5–19 year olds
- Working with schools, children, young people and families
- 'A day in the life of a school nurse'

Introduction

This book provides practical advice to school nurses using current literature to support the discussions. It is based on the experiences of school nurses across the United Kingdom (UK), who have contributed to the content. It considers the latest government plans for the development of school nursing practice and how this fits with the public health agenda. There are a number of case studies throughout the book based on real-life experiences to illustrate the issues. All names have been changed to protect anonymity throughout the book.

In 2011, the Department of Health (DH) initiated a review of the contribution that school nurses make to the Healthy Child Programme (HCP) and a model of school nursing practice was developed (DH, 2012a) (see Figure 1.1).

Key knowledge and skills were identified and highlighted as crucial to the 'unique selling point' for school nurses – vital given the commissioning agenda and the changes to health and social care made by the coalition Government which came into power in May 2010. The new proposed structure to NHS England sees the planned abolition of Primary Care Trusts and the establishment of local

↑ Developing the services for an effective Healthy Child Programme 5–19

'The Offer'

Your community has a range of health services (including GP and community services) for children, young people and their families. School nurses develop and provide these and make sure you know about them.

Universal services from your school nurse team provide the Healthy Child Programme to ensure a healthy start for every child (e.g. Public Health, including immunisations and health checks). They support children and parents to ensure access to a range of community services.

Universal plus delivers a swift response from your school nurse service when you need specific expert help e.g. with sexual health, mental health concerns, long-term health issues and additional health needs.

Universal partnership plus delivers ongoing support from your school nurse team from a range of local services working together with you to deal with more complex issues over a period of time (e.g. with voluntary and community organisations and your local authority).

Services and pathways
Services led by qualified school nurse and delivered in a range of settings:
■ School
■ Other education settings
■ Primary care
■ Youth and community
■ Home and residential settings

Developing pathways
■ Transition from health visiting to school nursing
■ Complex needs (school setting)
■ Safeguarding (including domestic violence and sexual exploitation)
■ Youth justice

* Additional pathways may include: Looked After Children, young carers and Child and Adolescent Mental Health Services

Quality standards
The service provided should encapsulate the 'You're Welcome' Quality Criteria
■ Accessibility
■ Publicity
■ Confidentiality and consent
■ Environment
■ Staff training, skills, attitudes and values
■ Joined-up working
■ Young people's involvement in monitoring and evaluation of patient experience
■ Health issues for young people
■ Sexual and reproductive health services
■ Specialist and targeted child and adolescent mental health services

DH 2011, British Youth Council 2011

← Safeguarding →

Figure 1.1 School nursing for improved health and wellbeing for children and young people

2

↑ Developing the services for an effective Healthy Child Programme 5–19 ↑

> **Public Health White Paper Update and Next Steps**
> Professionals such as health visitors and school nurses will have a role in helping to develop local approaches to public health, provide links between public health and the NHS and leadership in promoting good health and addressing inequalities.

> ***Outcomes: leading & contributing to:**
> ■ Improved health and wellbeing and a reduction in health inequalities.
> ■ Promoted healthy lifestyles and social cohesion by reaching and influencing the wider community.
> ■ Improved planning of local services to reduce health inequalities
>
> **Success measures: school nurses leading & contributing to 'healthy, happy children and young people'**
> ■ Increased access to evidence-based interventions through the Healthy Child Programme to children and families and tailored to specific need.
> ■ Young people reporting a high level of satisfaction and clinical effectiveness with school nursing service.
> ■ Reduced numbers of children requiring formal safeguarding arrangements – achieved through early identification and intervention.
> ■ Increased public health work to promote healthy lifestyles and social cohesion.
> ■ Increased uptake of early help and access to evidence based preventative services, which are tailored to meet individual and family needs, including support for parental needs e.g. mental health concerns.
> ■ Increased uptake from children, young people and families, of preventative services tailored to their needs and all families access evidence-based programmes.
> ■ Reduction in school absence due to poor health and/or additional health needs or complex needs.
> ■ Improved mental health and wellbeing including reduced bullying.
> ■ Improved co-ordination of training delivered to school staff to support pupils with complex health and/or additional needs.
> ■ Reduced incidences of obesity and positive lifestyle changes through improved coverage of National Child Measuring Programme.
> ■ Children and young people feel supported and able to make positive changes to their health and wellbeing.
> ■ Reduction in prevalence of chlamydia in 15–24 year olds and reduction in under 18 year olds conception rates.
> ■ Reduction in proportion of young people who frequently use illicit drugs or alcohol or that smoke.

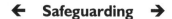

← Safeguarding →

Figure 1.1 *(continued)*

Developing the profession to lead and deliver seamless services for children, young people and families

The unique role of the school nursing service:

Delivering public health services to children and young people should be led by a Specialist Community Public Health Nurse (SCPHN) supported by a team with an appropriate skill mix to reflect local need. The school nursing service will improve children and young people's health and wellbeing by:

■ Leading, delivering and evaluating universal Public Health programmes for school-aged children and young people, both within school and community settings.

■ Taking an evidence based approach to delivering cost effective programmes or interventions which contribute to children and young people's health and wellbeing e.g. reductions in childhood obesity and under 18-year-old conception rates.

■ Referring and delegating within the team to maximise resources and utilise expertise of other skilled professionals.

■ Supporting seamless transition into school, from primary to secondary school and transition into adulthood.

■ Leading support for children and young people with complex and/or additional health needs including education, training and support for families, carers and school staff.

■ Identifying children and young people in need of early help and where appropriate providing support to improve their life chances and prevent abuse and neglect. This includes working with children and young people at risk of becoming involved in gangs or youth violence;

■ Contributing as part of a multi-agency team, to support children, young people and families, particularly those with multiple needs;

■ Supporting vulnerable children including children in care and support for their carers (including young people in contact with Youth Justice system).

Skills:
■ Graduate workforce;
■ Clinical;
■ Leadership;
■ Partnership and collaborative working;
■ Communication and negotiation;
■ Coaching and mentoring;
■ Children and young people Public Health specialist, skilled in:
  – Assessment;
  – Needs analysis and population data;
  – Evaluation and review;
  – Developing and implementing care plans.

Knowledge
■ Outcome-focused approaches;
■ Experts for wider health and wellbeing; for prevention and public health; for building family and community capacity.

Figure 1.1 *(continued)*

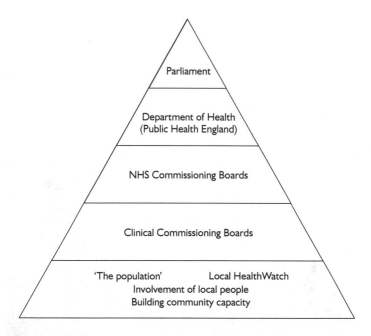

Figure 1.2 The proposed structure of the NHS in England (2011).

Clinical Commissioning Groups (CCGs), with the NHS Commissioning Board overseeing and organising the commissioning framework (Figure 1.2).

The commissioning framework will focus on the productivity of services, where productivity may be defined as the 'measure of the efficiency of the product'. The 'product' in the NHS, one could argue, is improved health outcomes for individuals. The aims of the public health outcomes framework (DH, 2012b) are to increase healthy life expectancy and reduce the differences in healthy life expectancy across communities (i.e. reduce inequalities). These are not new public health aims and school nurses have been contributing to this agenda for many years, the difference is that they will need to be able to demonstrate the effectiveness of what they do (see Chapter 7).

A common theme running through national policy in health, public health, education and social care is the devolvement of responsibility for services to local areas (DH, 2012b). This has both positive and negative consequences. It enables local areas to interpret guidelines according to the needs of the local population, but it also means that 'standardised services' are less likely across the country. The school nurse development programme attempts to offer a standardised service that still provides a flexible service to children and young people according to local need (DH, 2012a).

The school nurse role has become specialised following the introduction of the third part of the register and the production of the four domains, 10 principles and 24 standards of proficiency (Nursing and Midwifery Council [NMC], 2004) (see Box 1.1).

Box 1.1 The four domains, 10 principles and 24 standards of proficiency

Domain A – The search for health needs

A1 – Surveillance and assessment of the population's health and wellbeing.

A1.1 Collect and structure data and information on the health and wellbeing and related needs of a defined population.

A1.2 Analyse, interpret and communicate data and information on the health and wellbeing and related needs of a defined population.

A1.3 Develop and sustain relationships with groups and individuals with the aim of improving health and social wellbeing.

A1.4 Identify individuals, families and groups who are at risk and in need of further support.

A1.5 Undertake screening of individuals and populations and respond appropriately to findings.

Domain B – Stimulation of awareness of health needs

B1 – Collaborative working for health and wellbeing.

B1.1 Raise awareness about health and social wellbeing and related factors, services and resources.

B1.2 Develop, sustain and evaluate collaborative work.

B2 – Working with, and for communities to improve health and wellbeing.

B2.1 Communicate with individuals, groups and communities about promoting their health and wellbeing.

B2.2 Raise awareness about the actions that groups and individuals can take to improve their health and social wellbeing.

B2.3 Develop capacity and confidence of individuals and groups, including families and communities, to influence and use available services, information and skills, acting as advocate where appropriate.

B2.4 Work with others to protect the public's health and wellbeing from specific risks.

Domain C – Influences on policies affecting health

C1 – Developing health programmes and services and reducing inequalities.

C1.1 Work with others to plan implement and evaluate programmes to improve health and wellbeing.

C1.2 Identify and evaluate service provision and support networks for individual's families and groups in the local area or setting.

C2 – Policy and strategic development and implementation to improve health and wellbeing.

C2.1 Appraise policies and recommend changes to improve health and wellbeing.

C2.2 Interpret and apply health and safety legislation and approve codes of practice with regard for the environment, wellbeing and protection of those who work with the wider community.

C2.3 Contribute to policy development.

C2.4 Influence policies affecting health.

C3 – Research and development to improve health and wellbeing.

C3.1 Develop implement and evaluate and improve practice on the basis of research evidence and evaluation.

Domain D – Facilitation of health enhancing activities

D1 – Promoting and protecting the population's health and wellbeing.

D1.1 Work in partnership with others to prevent the occurrence of needs and risks relating to health and wellbeing.

D1.2 Work in partnership with others to protect the public's health and wellbeing from specific risks.

D2 – Developing quality and risk management within an evaluative culture.

D2.1 Prevent, identify and minimise risk of interpersonal abuse or violence safeguarding children and other vulnerable people initiating the management of cases involving actual or potential abuse or violence where needed.

D3 – Strategic leadership for health and wellbeing.

D3.1 Apply leadership skills and manage projects to improve health and wellbeing.

D3.2 Plan, deliver and evaluate programmes to improve the health and wellbeing of individuals and groups.

D4 – Ethically manage self, people and resources to improve health and wellbeing.

D4.1 Manage teams, individuals and resources ethically and effectively.

There has been an enduring misconception that the school nurse works in a school and only undertakes first-aid and checks attendance registers. The qualified Specialist Community Public Health Nurse (SCPHN) role is very different. These nurses work as a leader of the school health team delivering the Healthy Child Programme (5–19 years) across a diverse range of settings (DH/Department for Children Schools and Families [DCSF], 2009). There are different models of practice across the country and some nurses are based in mainstream schools or special schools while others are based in the community. Qualified SCPHNs have been specifically trained to a minimum of degree level and have specialist knowledge that enables them to contribute to the four domains of public health practice (DH, 2012b):

- Improve the wider determinants of health
- Health improvement
- Health protection
- Healthcare, public health and preventing premature mortality

Research was done in 2011 by the British Youth Council (BYC) to contribute to the school nurse development plan. It found that many young people had not had experience of their school nurse, but those that had valued the experience:

> Nearly three quarters of young people (73%) haven't visited their school nurse for anything other than immunisations. Yet those who had visited their school nurse told BYC that they have had a very positive experience – eight out of ten said their school nurse was approachable and friendly. Young people think more pupils need to know that their school nurse can provide advice on top teen health worries and help young people before they reach 'crisis point'.

> Young people want their school nurse to become a familiar face in their school. At the moment, nearly half are unsure who their school nurse is. All schools in England do have a school nurse who visits their school to offer care, advice and treatment; often one school nurse will work with several primary and secondary schools (BYC, 2011).

This chapter gives an overview of some of the issues around working in the community as a public health practitioner and considers the challenges of leading the Healthy Child Programme (HCP) (DH/DCSF, 2009). A key question is how work can be prioritised given the potential workload of the school health teams across the country. The subsequent chapters in the book will explore more fully the role of the school nurse:

The development of school nursing practice

Florence Nightingale suggested in the 19th century that nursing should be concerned with public health and improving the conditions which impact on health (Nightingale, 1860). School nursing arose out of a need to improve the conditions of children at a time of health and social reform during the Victorian era (BBC, 2010). The emphasis on public health and health promotion introduced by Florence Nightingale has laid the foundations for specialist community public health nursing practice today (Nightingale, 1860). The Manchester and Salford Reform Association was established in 1852, following closely on from the 1848 Public Health Act. This introduced 'sanitary visitors' to the evolving public health agenda and their initial role was didactic, giving information to families on issues of hygiene, food and standards of cleanliness in the home. They later became known as health visitors and Florence Nightingale set up the first training courses in Buckinghamshire in 1890 (Robothom and Frost, 2005). The first school nurses emerged at the same time, with a role in gathering information in the school setting, but it was not until the start of the 20th century that the school health service was formally established. Until 1944, school nursing and health visiting were closely linked with the same training, the distinction between them being through the authority by which they were employed. The 1944 Education Act made the distinction that:

> The nursing staff consists of a number of nurses under a senior or nursing superintendent.

> These, for the most part, act as school nurses under the education authority and as health visitors under the public health authority, and a Regulation recently made under the Education Act, 1944, is to the effect that every nurse to be appointed by the education authority for the purpose of the school health service shall possess the qualification prescribed for a health visitor... (Underwood, 1946)

History shows that the career trajectory of health visiting from then was very different from that of school nursing. The following decades saw school nurses as largely the handmaidens of the school medical officers and their role continued to be one of inspection and screening. Screening for head lice became a key memory in the minds of many children growing up during the 1950s and 1960s and one which endures even today, much to the frustration of many school nurses (Wright, 2011).

There have been many changes to the role of school nurses over the last few decades. Like other areas of nursing practice, they have become professional, autonomous practitioners who lead teams to promote the health and wellbeing of school-age children. Today, there are few school medical officers involved in school health, and school nurses have moved away from a medical model to a broader approach encompassing a variety of disciplines. Their training came into line with other community nurses in 1984 and their role is continuing to evolve; they have both an important public health role and a clinical role one which sets them apart from other health professionals (Wright, 2011).

Some newly-qualified school nurses will have worked as community staff nurses before qualification, and therefore have insight into the challenges of working in the community setting. Others may not have worked in that environment before and will have come from a range of nursing backgrounds into school nursing. Whatever their background, the role of a qualified school nurse is one that requires specific knowledge, skills and attitudes in order to lead teams in promoting child public health. A diversity of backgrounds for school nurses is invaluable to the service and those coming from all three branches of the nursing profession – child, adult and mental health – have a contribution to make to the role and to school health teams.

The key responsibilities of the school nurse have evolved across the UK in response to local need and the role varies across the country. However, it is also important to ensure that the key roles and responsibilities are clearly defined. The school nurse development programme (SNDP) *Getting it Right for Children, Young People and Their Families* (DH, 2012a) provides a clear model for future school nursing practice, with an emphasis on leadership and child public health. School nurses form a key part of the school health team and must work within a broader community in order to effectively promote the health of children and young people.

How can building partnerships promote positive health and wellbeing?

Building partnerships is crucial to the role of school nurses, particularly given limited resources. The number of connections that school nurses make will impact on their ability to reach groups that are most vulnerable and in need of services and therefore, on their ability to contribute to reducing inequalities. They are identified as leaders and, as such, need to be at the forefront of developing sustainable local public health services; they cannot work alone in achieving this. They will work with a wide range of groups, including statutory and voluntary services as well as local communities.

School nurses work within a multidisciplinary team and should be aware of who they work most closely with in order to act in the best interests of children, young people and their families. As well as working with communities, parents, carers, children and young people, there are a wide range of professionals with whom the school nurse will come into contact with. Here are just a few:

- **General practitioners (GPs)**: The relationship with GPs varies across the country. Some school nurses are based in GP surgeries, which means that they have clear access and good communication links with them. Those who are not based in GP surgeries should endeavour to make strong links, particularly around sharing information about specific children and families (see 'A day in the life of a school nurse'– p. 32).
- **Health visitors**: Theoretically, school nurses work most closely with health visitors. Their training is the same, with the same standards of competencies which are applied to the under-fives. The Healthy Child Programme includes recommendations for good communication with and transitions between health visitors and the school health teams.
- **Teachers**: A good relationship with teachers is essential for the foundation of good, multi-agency working. Referrals from teachers form a cornerstone of school nurse practice. The head of PSHE is also an important link.
- **Head teachers**: It is important to have good links to the head of a school. No changes or initiatives can be introduced without their cooperation.
- **School governors**: Projects such as setting up health drop-ins will require the support of school governors.
- **Special educational needs coordinators (SENCOs)**: A health input to statements of special needs is important.
- **Speech and language teams (SALT)**
- **Audiology staff**
- **Community paediatricians**
- **Child and Adolescent Mental Health Services (CAMHS)**
- **Social Services**
- **Community children's nurses**
- **Dietitians**

- **Hospital staff**
- **Educational welfare officers/Education social workers**
- **Youth services including youth offending services**
- **Voluntary agencies**
- **The wider community**

Building community capacity

School nurses have a role to play in working with local communities to improve health and wellbeing; this is explicit in the NMC competencies (Box 1.1). The term 'capacity building' originates from work done worldwide in developing communities, where it is deemed important to build the skills and competencies of local people to sustain themselves rather than rely on aid from other countries (United Nations Development Programme [UNDP], 2012). This concept is now used in other contexts, and in the UK, building community capacity is about utilising individuals, groups, organisations and networks in projects that are identified through local needs assessments. This is an important way to use or develop the skills and competencies of local people in addressing a community issue and may be crucial given finite resources. There are a number of advantages to building community capacity, including issues around the sustainability of projects. Projects which have been generated and developed locally are more likely to succeed over time, and this relates to the investment that individuals or groups have in the project. This may be an emotional investment, where people feel strongly about a problem or issue and are prepared to give their time, knowledge, skills or expertise to improve a situation. A good example of this is the aftermath of the riots in London in the summer of 2011, where local communities united to help others.

Other examples of community projects include:

- Supporting and training parents to set up local parenting groups
- Setting up drop-in advice services for parents, children and young people
- Working to address alcohol-related problems in local areas
- Working with the community to address anti-social behaviour and crime
- Working with young people who are excluded from school
- Setting up sexual health services in rural areas
- Contributing to support groups for children and young people with specific needs

Critical to forming good partnerships are clear lines of communication and awareness of the network of groups in local areas. Newly-qualified school nurses should start to build a resource and contact pack that will enable them to build a directory of professionals, local services and community groups which they can utilise to build community capacity. It is also good practice to take the opportunity early in the role to make time for an introductory visit to different professionals and agencies – this may be valuable later.

Autonomous decision-making

Although school nurses work as part of the multidisciplinary team, they are also responsible for autonomous decisions. As qualified nurses of course, school nurses work to a code of conduct (NMC, 2008) and are accountable for their actions. They therefore work within a professional framework which protects the public, but also gives definition to the autonomous decision-making processes. In addition to this, local frameworks for working with children, young people and families are also in place with specific guidelines, protocols and procedures. These should be available and accessible in all school health team bases and new staff should be made aware of them at induction.

Working in the community means having to make independent, informed decisions, but this should not mean the same as making isolated decisions. School nurses and their teams need to be supported in the decisions they make by regular training, team meetings, clinical supervision and appraisals. It is the responsibility of all school nurses to ensure that they are up to date with their practice and to raise concerns if they feel unsupported. The first year in practice for newly-qualified school nurses can be a stressful time and they should be supported by preceptors (NMC, 2006). School nurses who have undertaken the degree qualification have demonstrated competence in the four domains of specialist community public health nursing (SCPHN) (NMC, 2004). This means that they have specific training in working with individuals and groups and work to a public health agenda. School nurses are accountable to their professional body, but they are also accountable to the schools, managers, colleagues, parents and children within their sphere of work. Qualified SCPHNs have the knowledge to develop the skills of making decisions with young people which is based on four fundamental ethical principles (Nuffield Council on Bioethics, 2007):

- Beneficence – to do good
- Non-maleficence – the 'no harm' principle
- Respect for autonomy – understanding the need for choices balanced against acting in the best interests of children and young people
- Justice for all – considering the broader implications to others when decisions are made

Decisions are not always easy and school nurses can consider the balance of these four principles to help them make appropriate decisions which promote the health of children and young people. Decision-making skills are discussed further in Chapter 3. The code of conduct is a key source of guidance for school nurses (NMC, 2008).

What risks should school nurses be aware of in the community?

School nurses can be classed as 'mobile workers working away from their fixed base' (Health and Safety Executive [HSE], 2009, p. 2). There are two main pieces of legislation that should protect workers in this situation.

The Health and Safety at Work Act 1974: Section 2 sets out a duty of care on employers to ensure the health, safety and welfare of their employees whilst they are at work.

The Management of Health and Safety at work Regulations 1999: Regulation 3 states that every employer shall make a suitable and sufficient assessment of:

■ the risks to the health and safety of his employees to which they are exposed whilst they are at work; and
■ the risks to the health and safety of persons not in his employment arising out of or in connection with the conduct by him of his undertaking

Employers have a responsibility to ensure their employees' safety, and all local areas will have guidelines and policies around working in the community. This is based on a risk assessment for these types of workers and this should be available to all staff in their bases. It is important that there is an induction for new members of staff to clarify these procedures.

Personal safety

There are some common sense approaches to personal safety such as:

■ Tell someone where you are going and when you will return and keep them informed if there is a change of plan.
■ Keep a mobile phone on, charged and accessible at all times (on silent if necessary).
■ Have a separate work mobile and don't give out personal numbers.
■ Keep car keys accessible if visiting people in their own home.
■ Make sure you have easy access to the exit.
■ Don't visit known problem families on your own.
■ Ensure that you are fully aware of any individual school policies.

■ Consider any consent issues when talking to children and young people (this is discussed later in Chapters 3 and 6).

Violence and aggression

There are personal risks as a professional in any setting and there will always be the potential to be hurt in any situation. It can be particularly problematic in the community because school nurses may be dealing with difficult situations, such as child protection, domestic violence and confidential information. Anger, fear, anxiety and frustration can lead normally rational people to behave in an unpredictable way. This may include aggressive behaviour. Understanding how to defuse situations is important and the ability to read the early verbal and non-verbal cues that alert you to a problem is crucial. This means that good communication skills are essential and they have been a fundamental part of nurse training for some time. In the community, these skills need to be particularly developed and the ability to negotiate and manage conflict is explored in Chapter 2.

Intimidation

Individuals and parents in particular can become intimidating if they feel threatened or undermined. School nurses may be talking in confidence to young people about personal problems that they are not obliged to talk to parents about (see the Fraser guidelines in Chapter 6). This has the potential for parents to become very angry (see Case study 1.1).

Case study 1.1

Anna, a 15-year-old girl at an upper school, tells the school nurse that she is pregnant and a pregnancy test confirms this. Anna says that she thinks she is about 16 weeks pregnant. The school nurse discusses the options with her, encouraging her to talk to her parents. However, Anna states clearly that she does not want to talk to her mother as 'she would kill me'. Anna says she wants a termination and the school nurse again discusses the options with her and gives her relevant contacts at the British Pregnancy Advisory Service. Anna comes back the following week. Anna has not approached anyone about a termination and the school nurse has the feeling that Anna wants to keep the baby but is frightened of her mother. The dilemma for the school nurse is maintaining confidentiality while protecting Anna's safety. The decision is taken out of the school nurse's hands when Anna's

> friend tells Anna's mother about the pregnancy. The mother is very angry and comes into school threatening both the school nurse and the school. She has to be escorted off the premises. The mother also continues to threaten the school nurse through the health centre. The school and the school nurse's manager fully support the school nurse as she has followed clear guidelines in this case and the mother is threatened with legal action. The threatening behaviour then ceases.
>
> Anna is persuaded by the mother to have a late termination of pregnancy.

School nurses need to be very clear about the policy on aggression, violence and intimidation and never give personal details to any child, young person or their family. Some areas, recognising the value of Information Technology (IT), use text messaging services or emails as a valuable means of communicating with young people. This must be done in a professional way at work rather than at home, and local protocols must protect individuals from harm.

What are the health and safety issues around immunisation in schools?

Working with Patient Group Directives

Nurses working on the immunisation programmes work with Patient Group Directives (PGDs). These are group prescriptions signed by a local committee/panel of senior nurses, doctors and pharmacists and relate to a defined group of people. Those who are eligible to administer the immunisations are listed within the group prescription and this is regularly updated. Regular training and updating for school nurses should be part of continuing professional development (see Chapter 2).

PGDs can be provided for other drugs, such as emergency contraception, which may be necessary for school nurses providing sexual health services. Some training education establishments have introduced the community nurse prescribing course within the degree programme, enabling school nurses to prescribe drugs from a community formula. This has some limitations and other school nurses undertake the non-medical prescribing course as part of their continuing professional development. This is dependent on local needs and local agreements.

Infection control

All nurses need to be aware of the principles of infection control. Standard infection control precautions need to be applied to all work that school nurses do and in particular, in clinical work such as immunisation. Local areas have guidelines on infection control, and the fundamental issues for school nurses include:

- Hand hygiene: alcohol-based hand rub should be available for staff in the absence of effective hand-washing facilities.
- The use of personal protective equipment: there should be clear local guidelines on the use of protective equipment, such as wearing gloves at immunisation sessions. This should be based on a risk assessment.
- The safe use and disposal of sharps: no immunisations should be given without correctly assembled sharps boxes.
- Education of healthcare personnel and also other staff including school staff. Schools may seek advice from the school nurse about infection control.
- School nurses may be consulted about childhood infectious diseases by schools or parents and there should be clarity about whether children should be excluded from school. The Health Protection Agency provides the most up to date information on infectious diseases in schools and other childcare settings (HPA, 2011). It is important to maintain currency about this, as recommendations change from time to time. Fundamentally, if a child or young person is acutely unwell, one should question whether they should be in school.
- The spread of communicable/notifiable diseases. School nurses may be involved when there is an outbreak of a communicable disease such as tuberculosis. They may be required to screen populations for the disease and implement immunisation programmes if needed.

The National Institute for Health and Clinical Excellence also provides guidelines on infection control (NICE, 2003). These guidelines are due to be updated in 2012.

The safe storage and transport of vaccines

The maintenance of the cold chain and clear protocols about the collection and return of vaccines should be part of the school nurse training in practice and regularly updated (see Chapter 2).

What are the professional responsibilities of the school nurse?

Political awareness (commissioning services, research and development)

Qualified school nurses need to be politically aware both in the broadest sense of monitoring change to government policy and also with regard to local politics. School nurses should be confident about their contribution to a wide range of public health issues and crucially, be active in creating opportunities to raise the school nurse profile in order to deliver the Healthy Child Programme (HCP) for school-age children. Skill in 'selling the service' to commissioners is important and the ability to demonstrate the effectiveness of the uniqueness of school health interventions is vital. This is discussed further in later chapters. The Wanless report into the cost of the NHS in 2004 established a need to demonstrate the effectiveness of interventions (Wanless, 2004). The findings remain significant and are reflected in the development of school nursing and also within the HCP. Qualified school nurses must be prepared to lead the way forward in fighting to increase resources to achieve good health for all.

A quick guide to the political process

- **Green Papers**: these are consultation papers before a White Paper is produced. There are opportunities here to contribute to and comment on government policy.
- **White Papers**: produced normally following the Green Paper once consultation has occurred. White Papers are produced to publicly announce government policy on an issue, and they may be a prelude to passing a law or forming part of a bill. There may still be opportunities to contribute or to make amendments or updates.
- **Bills and legislation**: these set out a proposal either for a new law or for an update of a current law. They can be instigated by either the House of Commons or the House of Lords and must go through both houses before they can be approved. There are several stages to the process: a first reading, second reading, committee stage, report stage and third reading. These stages are repeated in both houses and then go to a consideration of amendments. The final stage is the Royal Assent. Most bills are initiated by government, but private members' bills can also be introduced. However, these rarely become law.
- **Acts of Parliament**: once a bill has Royal Assent, it is 'enacted' (becomes law). This is no longer guidance, but has to be acted upon. If successive governments want to change any law, they have to go through this process again.

Protocols and policies

School nurses need to be aware of, and contribute to, community protocols and policies. This needs to be both on a local level, such as policies around child protection, immunisation or developing care pathways, and also nationally. It is important for school nurses to maintain currency in their work by using the best available evidence. This means keeping up to date with the most current thinking on a range of issues. Consultation documents from the government are regularly advertised by the nursing press and on government websites, and school nurses need to keep informed in order for them to contribute. It is important to maintain the profile of school nurses, and this can only be achieved by making sure their voice is heard. The school nurse development programme recognised this and disseminated information for consultation across the UK to many different stakeholders. The Department of Health called for evidence of good practice from practitioners, which was distributed through the main stakeholders in the school nurse development group. The development of research skills is explored further in Chapter 2.

Some useful websites to regularly visit are:

■ The Department of Health [DH]: http://www.dh.gov.uk/
■ The Department for Education [DE]: http://www.education.gov.uk/
■ The Chief Nursing Officer Bulletin [CNO]: http://cno.dh.gov.uk/category/school-nursing/
■ The Centre for Excellence and Outcomes for Children and Young People's Services [C4EO]: http://www.c4eo.org.uk/
■ Children & Young People Now: http://www.cypnow.co.uk/
■ The British Youth Council [BYC]: http://www.byc.org.uk/
■ NHS evidence: https://www.evidence.nhs.uk/qipp#

Delivering the Healthy Child Programme (HCP) for 5–19-year-olds

The coalition government in 2011 made a commitment to the Healthy Child Programme (HCP). The *HCP from 5 to 19* (DH/DCSF 2009) is aimed at young people from 5 years up to their 20th birthday. As with the *Healthy Child Programme: pregnancy and the first five years of life*, it considers *universal* and *progressive services*. Universal services refer to what all children need (such as immunisations) and progressive services are those which target those with specific health needs. The HCP originated from the *Every Child Matters* agenda introduced by the Labour government in 2004 (DH/DfES, 2004). Other drivers for the programme came from: *Health for All Children* (Hall and Elliman, 2003), and the *National Service Framework for Children, Young People and Maternity Services* (DH, 2004a).

The key points of the HCP are:

- Early intervention
- Safeguarding
- Preventative public health programmes
- Identification of need
- Appropriate services and referrals
- Working together
- Minimising inequality

What does the HCP recommend?

Recommended schedule: 5–11 years (universal services)

1. Information sharing between health visitors (HV) and school health and education on school entry. This will include information on developmental needs.
2. A health assessment including reviewing immunisation status, dental health and a height, weight, vision and hearing check. Height and weight are also reviewed as part of the National Child Measurement Programme (NCMP).
3. Support for emotional health and wellbeing for children and their families. School health teams can contribute to Social and Emotional Aspects of Learning (SEAL) in the school and also the Healthy Schools Initiatives. This may include contributing to the personal, social and health education programme in the school.
4. Support the Change4life campaign with regard to healthy eating and encourage this in the school setting (Change4life, 2012).
5. Consider aspects of physical activity and advise schools and parents on the healthy weight of children and young people. School nurses may contribute to the healthy schools initiatives.
6. Safeguarding and child protection as per *Working Together to Safeguard Children* (HM Government, 2006).
7. Use of the Common Assessment Framework (CAF) is recommended within the HCP and development of the Team Around the Child (TAC) for children identified with specific needs. School nurses are potential lead professionals for this work.
8. There should be a clear referral route for the school following any identified need through the school health team to more specialised services such as

CAMHS. The development of care pathways has been established in many areas.

9. Information and support should be available for parents through various means: through the school health team, HCP websites, school websites or NHS Choices.

Recommended schedule: 5–11 years (progressive services)

1. Immunisations for children at risk. Check immunisation status and refer if necessary.
2. Supporting emotional health, psychological wellbeing and mental health. Targeted Mental Health in Schools (TaMHS) services can be accessed if available. Consideration of primary, targeted and specialist services (Tiers 2, 3 and 4) for those children at risk of mental health problems. Again, clear referral routes and responsibilities should be clarified by the school health team. Drop-in services for children and parents are established in some areas of the country.
3. Overweight and obese children. Advice, support, signposting and referral on to secondary services if necessary. There are projects being run by school nurses such as MEND (Mind Exercise, Nutrition, Do it) or the equivalent.
4. The child in need. Responsibility for the assessment of need in the CAF and TAC as the lead professional.
5. Health assessments for the looked after child (LAC). Local Authorities are required to ensure that a Strengths and Difficulties Questionnaire is completed for all their looked after children. School nurses may be involved in health assessments with good opportunities to support looked after children and promote health and help foster parents fill in these questionnaires.
6. Children with special educational needs. Health advice is required within the assessment of children with special educational needs. School nurses are available to schools to coordinate these health assessments.
7. Children with complex health needs should have a comprehensive care plan coordinated by the school health team. Care pathways can be developed to support children with particular needs (see Chapter 2). Policies should be in place to manage medicines in schools and school staff trained accordingly (see Chapter 2).
8. Support for young carers through the school health team.
9. Other support for parents and carers. The school nurse should be aware of specific projects that are set up to help families in need. This will be crucial with limited resources and it is important to signpost families to projects and

make sure that these projects know who the school nurse is. Such projects will vary across the country but may include family intervention projects; family support workers through the Children's Centres; and parenting intervention programmes. Many projects are run by charities such as Action for Children. School nurses should be involved in detailed community profiling to understand clearly what is available in their area.

10. Support for parents with specific needs such as drug and alcohol problems, mental health problems, learning difficulties or families where there is domestic violence. School nurses should again be aware of available specialist services and referral routes and be clear about safeguarding and child protection procedures.

Recommended schedule: 11–16 years (universal)

1. A health review in year 7 (11–12 years). Some areas have developed a review process at the transition to secondary school which involves administering and reviewing questionnaires. The purpose of this is to review immunisation status, alert the school nurse to any health problems and also to highlight the role of the school nurse to young people entering secondary school.
2. Immunisation programmes (HPV and school leavers' boosters).
3. Support for emotional health, psychological wellbeing and mental health. School nurses can contribute to PSHE programmes effectively to promote positive relationships and emotional wellbeing (see Chapter 5).
4. Promoting healthy weights as with the 5–11 schedule.
5. Sexual health and wellbeing. Local Authorities and the NHS are expected to work together to provide accessible, confidential services for sexual health using the *You're Welcome* framework (see Chapter 6).
6. Ongoing support for children in need as with the 5–11 schedule. Includes safeguarding issues and consideration of additional needs.

Recommended schedule: 11–16 years (progressive services)

1. Emotional health, psychological wellbeing and mental health. Many secondary schools now have a drop-in service for young people to access one-to-one support and advice at Tiers 1 and 2 CAMHS. School nurses lead these programmes and should work in partnership with CAMHS to ensure good referral routes. School nurses also need training in targeted and specialist services (Tiers 3 and 4), i.e. when to refer. It will also be important to have regular clinical supervision with specialist CAMHS (see Chapter 3).

2. Young people at risk from a range of problems such as drugs, alcohol, smoking or obesity should be supported within the school, with school nurses acting as gatekeepers for referrals to specialist services. Awareness of other agencies is crucial: for example the local drugs and alcohol teams and NHS stop smoking groups.

3. Looked after children. Adolescents need further support through this stage of development as there is evidence of poor outcomes and risk-taking behaviours. School nurses are well positioned to give advice on both emotional and physical needs through health assessments at this stage.

4. Young people with special educational needs. The transition into adulthood and the workplace needs to be managed within a multidisciplinary team.

5. Young people with complex health needs also need transitional support as they move into adult services.

6. Young people in contact with the youth justice system. These young people may need additional support to re-integrate into the education system and consider their healthcare needs in the event of custody.

Recommended schedule: 16–19 years (universal services)

1. Immunisation status check.

2. Young people entering further education. This group of young people are still in need of support for their own health and wellbeing. They may be at a vulnerable stage of development, and once they enter Further Education (FE) or Higher Education (HE) they may be susceptible to poor health and should be offered continuing support through the school health teams. This may be achieved through the Healthy FE programmes. The personal tutor systems may be an important link for the Healthy Child Programme teams.

3. Emotional health and wellbeing. Young people and their families should have access to psychological wellbeing and mental health support. School nurses may also be able to contribute to supporting the transitions that these young people make, particularly around moving from CAMHS to adult mental health services.

4. Sexual health services. Eighty per cent of under 18 conceptions are 16–17 year olds and many of these will be in the FE sector (DH/DCSF, 2009). Support for young people who have left school for FE should be ongoing and school nurses can contribute to this agenda. There may also be further opportunities to prepare young people more effectively for parenthood.

5. Physical activity. There is a drop out rate from physical activity among 16–19 year-olds. There is potential to work with young people through partnerships

with sports coordinators and voluntary agencies to maintain participation in sporting activities.

6. Ongoing support. All opportunities for offering health information should be taken at this age. This will include forming partnerships with professionals such as youth workers and social care.

7. Ongoing safeguarding responsibilities. This age range is recognised as problematic in terms of safeguarding. Teams need to be aware of the ongoing risks in this age group and offer support and advice through accessible services.

8. Support for parents. Parenting teenagers can also be problematic and parents may be experiencing real difficulties with setting boundaries and communicating with their adolescents. School nurses are in a good position to give support and advice.

Recommended schedule: 16–19 years (progressive services)

1. Immunisations for at-risk young people, as with the other age groups.

2. Emotional health, psychological wellbeing and mental health. Referral to specialised services for young people at risk. Clear understanding of the role of school nurses and clearly identified referral routes. Clinical supervision should be considered here with specialist services.

3. Drug and alcohol misuse. Consideration of local specialist services as well as support and advice through drop-ins. Also for consideration should be those leaving schools for FE and, later, HE.

4. Smoking cessation. Accessible support and referrals to NHS services if necessary.

5. Consideration of at-risk groups:
    (a) Looked after young people and the transition to FE and the workplace
    (b) Young people with complex welfare needs. May be ongoing from earlier ages.
    (c) Young people with special educational needs, as with the 11–16 age range. Consideration of the policy and procedures for the transition of young people from children's to adult health services: Transition: Moving on Well (DH/DCSF, 2008).
    (d) Young people with complex health needs. Consideration of the transitions and care planning should consider issues around accommodation and housing.
    (e) Young people leaving the care system. Care orders end at 18. Care leavers may need additional support to manage their own health needs. There is also evidence of young people leaving care at 16.

(f) One-to-one sexual health interventions for high-risk young people. NICE guidelines (2007) recommend that at-risk young people under 18 (for example, from disadvantaged backgrounds, those in care, and/or those who have low educational attainment) are offered one-to-one sexual health advice.

(g) Young people in contact with the youth justice system. There are school nurses in the country who have a dual role in the youth offending service and in school nursing.

(h) Support and advice for parents and carers: family pathfinders, Family Intervention Projects and Multi-Systemic Therapy (MST, 2011). MST is a community intervention for children and young people and their families where young people are at risk of offending behaviour. The scheme supports parenting capacity and works to increase young people's engagement with education, health and training to promote pro-social behaviours (MST, 2011).

A school health service is recommended in government policy, but is not a mandatory public health service. This means that commissioners have to make difficult decisions about the health and wellbeing of children and young people. Health and wellbeing boards will be responsible for identifying local need and planning services. The HCP has advice for commissioners where they are encouraged to:

Identify evidence-based interventions to address local needs (bearing in mind that implementing a programme well may be as important as choosing the right intervention) and

Identify currently provided services that are not supported by evidence and decide whether continued investment in these services is justified (HCP, p. 75)

The crucial message here is clear: that assessing need is vital and measuring the effectiveness of services is crucial. The school nurse role in this matter is discussed in Chapter 7.

School nurses need communication skills and particularly the ability to build relationships with a variety of professionals in order to deliver a service. The success of school nursing depends on both team and individual approaches to schools and, in particular, relationships with governors and head teachers, as they are leaders of individual schools. It seems logical to say that a 'healthy child' is more likely to achieve educationally and socially, and for school nurses, as public health practitioners, this is a top priority. Although health is a relative term, with many definitions, in this context, health is seen to mean the optimum health achievable given individual circumstances, such as disability, social deprivation, family dynamics or complex health needs. However, with the many demands on time in schools it is sometimes difficult to persuade others of this fundamental truth. Time and commitment are needed and qualified school nurses need to have a vision of what promoting the health of children and young people means in reality and how to market their service to relevant people and use finite resources efficiently and effectively. One also needs to add to this the cooperation of parents and young people themselves. Without their belief in their own health, a service is doomed to failure. As well as the schedule outlined above, Table 1.1 shows a summary of the diverse nature of the SN role.

Working with schools, children, young people and families

The school health team works in partnership with education to enable children to achieve in school. The evidence is clear that young people who do well in school are more likely to be employed, less likely to be anti-social and more likely to achieve economic wellbeing (Department for Education [DfE], 2010). Helping children and young people to stay healthy, given their individual circumstances, throughout their school life will give them the best chance of achieving this goal. This of course applies to both their physical and emotional health and wellbeing. A less altruistic view is that society has a collective responsibility to ensure a healthy workforce in order to maintain economic stability. This ultimate goal depends on partnerships with schools, children, young people, their families and local communities. School nurses are in a good position to form a link between agencies and act as advocates for children and young people.

Types of school

The way in which education is delivered in the UK has changed with the introduction of academies and free schools to the education system, and this may have an impact on school health teams. Academies were set up by the Labour government in 2000 and are publicly funded schools which operate outside of local authority control. The coalition government described them as independent, state-funded schools. Essentially, academies have more freedom than other state schools over their finances, the curriculum and teachers' pay and conditions. Legislation in 2011 allows primary, secondary and special schools to apply for academy status. They are established by sponsors from business, the voluntary sector or faith groups, and in theory work with the local community to provide a curriculum relevant

Table 1.1 The work of the school health team.

Potential area of work	Responsibility	Working with
Assessing need	Prioritising work as a team leader. Profiling area and schools to assess priorities	Schools, GP surgeries, public health, parents, children and young people
	Measuring outcomes	Other stakeholders
	Demonstrating need to local commissioning partners	National and local data
		Local quality measuring groups
		Commissioners
Assessing health risks	May need to give advice on health and safety issues at school and elsewhere – such as school trips. All schools have a health and safety policy	Health and safety executive. Planning care, medical needs in schools. Other statutory bodies
	Risk assessments on immunisation sessions or other specific work	Integrated teams Managers
Bullying	Supporting children, parents, teachers on bullying and contributing to bullying policies in schools	Schools, education, Local Authorities Other stakeholders
Child protection and children in need	Lead health professional for school-age child	Parents/carers/Social Services, education, police, voluntary sector and other relevant agencies
Children with chronic illness	Liaison and planning of care pathways	Community Children's Nurses, special schools, family, paediatricians, physiotherapists, occupational therapists
Children not in school	Screening, monitoring and support Contributing to care pathways	Travelling communities, educational social workers/welfare officers, METAS, PRUs, Local Authorities, home schooled children
Disability, special medical and educational needs	Support for parents and teachers for children with special medical and behavioural needs	Education, educational psychologists, learning support assistants, parents and teachers
Drop-ins	Work with others to provide convenient, confidential services to young people	Youth services, counselling services, sexual health services, voluntary sector

Table 1.1 (continued)

Potential area of work	Responsibility	Working with
Emotional health, psychological wellbeing and mental health Anxiety and stress Depression Loss and bereavement Divorce and separation Coping with transitions Low self-esteem	Drop-in work Recommended on-site support Tier 1/Tier 2 support May be multidisciplinary – may be in self-esteem groups- could be working with groups of parents Contribute to SEAL	CAMHS, Schools, GPs, parents, teachers, youth workers, youth offending teams, counsellors Multi-systems therapy projects
Enuresis	Lead for enuresis in some areas Develop care pathways	Parents/paediatricians/hospital or clinic staff/administration
Families with complex needs	Domestic violence, parents with alcohol or drugs problems, young carers	Family intervention programmes; young carers support, Social Services Multi-systems therapy projects
Hard to reach young people (or 'easy to ignore groups')	Consider young people not in school, education or employment (NEETS), homeless young people, those living in poverty, youth offenders, travelling families	Youth Offending services/Social Services/Local liaison groups/voluntary services/Education welfare officers
Health promotion	One-to-one, with PSHE programmes and opportunistic	Children, families, teachers and others
Immunisations	Lead for both routine immunisations and also for campaigns or outbreaks Also responsible for checking immunisation status at health reviews	Skill mix team may include nursery nurses, community staff nurses and administration staff Consider Patient Group Directives
Infection control; hygiene issues	Advice to schools on spread of infection; contributing to policy	Schools, families, HPA, infection control team. Report outbreaks
Looked after children (LAC)	Liaison with LAC nurses – medical assessments in schools or home	LAC nurse, school, family, paediatrician, GP, Social services
Parenting	Leading groups/training others to lead groups. Building community capacity	Parents, teachers
Personal, social and health education	Teaching in schools	Education, Healthy schools
'Political' action	Contribution to raising the profile of children's needs both in a local sense and also more broadly in central government – awareness of commissioning is crucial.	Working with health and social services, local authorities and schools Consultation documents (Green and White Papers)

Table 1.1 *(continued)*

Potential area of work	Responsibility	Working with
Policies and protocols	As team leader, ensure that policies and protocols are in place to protect the public (and staff)	Work with health and safety strategies to manage any risk
Research and development	Raise profile of school nurses – Create opportunities for research and publish research papers Contribute to research which demonstrates effectiveness of the school health service. Ensure dissemination of research appropriately.	Work with management and local authorities Cooperate with relevant journals to raise profile
Screening	Monitor ht/wt/vision/hearing on school entry. Health reviews as per HCP Child Health Measurement Programme	School, GPs, audiology, dietitians, SALT, orthoptist
Self-harming behaviour Substance misuse Cutting behaviour Attempted suicide	One-to-one work/drop-in services. PSHE	CAMHS, GPs, psychologists, drugs and alcohol action teams (DAAT), young persons substance misuse service provider, voluntary services such as AA, multi-systems therapy projects
Sexual health Pregnancy Sexually Transmitted Infection (STIs) Awareness of issues of sexual exploitation and vulnerability	Drop-in work; on site services are recommended Contribute to SRE programmes Chlamydia screening Free condom service	May involve teen pregnancy team and sexual health clinics, GP's, schools and governors 'You're Welcome' criteria Work with Fraser guidelines
Smoking	Consider both young people and parents; smoking advice and cessation groups The 3 A approach: Ask, Advise and Act	Parents, young people, GPs, smoking cessation groups, NHS services
Transitional support	Consider young people moving schools, dealing with loss, moving into adult services who have particular health or social needs Moving out of care at 18 Moving into further education.	Work with voluntary agencies, local authorities, other health professionals, schools Access to personal data Further Education colleges Higher Education Institutions
Weight management programmes such as MEND	Some areas take the lead, in others there is a referral process	Parents, schools, dietitians

to the area. The overall intention is to allow schools to be more autonomous and independent. An academy normally specialises in one or two areas (such as sports) and it is envisaged that, because they can create a specialised curriculum, they will serve to help regenerate disadvantaged communities by providing relevant programmes for the area (DfE, 2011).

In September 2011, 24 free schools opened. They are non-profit-making, independent state-funded schools. The intention is that they are set up by interested local people, such as teachers, businesses, universities or parents. They can be set up in appropriate community buildings, not necessarily in traditional school buildings. Anyone can apply to set up a free school and plans are approved by the Secretary of State for Education. They still come under the inspection of the Office for Standards in Education, Children's Services and Skills (Ofsted), and it is envisaged that they could help to solve the problem of a lack of school places in particular areas.

How these new schools will impact on the school health team is yet to be assessed, but it may be viewed as an opportunity to influence the curriculum in relation to personal health promotion. School nurses may want to be involved in the setting up of free schools in their areas.

Working with children and families in their own home or school setting

School nurses can see school-age children wherever they happen to be: in mainstream school, pupil referral units, special schools, at home, in community centres or in health centres. There are examples across the country of school nurses based in a secondary school (Chief Nursing Officer Bulletin [CNO], 2011). They function as community school nurses, but their base is on the school site. This is proving to be very effective and mirrors the New Labour target in 2004 that there should be one school nurse per secondary school and its feeder schools (DH, 2004b). Although this has been achieved in Wales, it had not been achieved in England in 2012.

A clear, cultural understanding of the school community and the area in which the school is situated is important in order to work within it. Individual school communities, however, may not always reflect the demographics of the local area, as children may come from some distance to attend a particular school (this may change if free schools become more common). This may be for a variety of reasons: it may be a faith school, an academy specialising in a particular subject or a grammar school. Schools have their own admissions criteria, which may not be that the pupil lives in the near locality. Whatever the differences, schools provide a potential for children and young people to have convenient, confidential access to a health professional for advice and information.

Working one-to-one with children and young people

Seeing young people on an individual basis gives opportunities to assess both individual need and also provide broader knowledge of the school curriculum with an opportunity to contribute to PSHE programmes (see Case study 1.2).

Case study 1.2

Two 15-year-old girls attended a newly-established drop-in service run by the school nurse, a local GP and a youth worker. They asked for information around sexual health and wanted to discuss contraception. During the conversation, it became clear that they had little understanding of sexual health and in particular the risks of contracting sexually transmitted infections. They both disclosed to the school nurse that they had very little information on this topic within the school curriculum and Personal, Health, Social and Economic education. The school nurse asked permission to approach the school, and the girls gave their consent. Following a meeting with the head teacher and the PSHE coordinator, the school nurse was able to contribute to the PSHE curriculum on sexual health throughout the school year. This also gave opportunities for the school nurse to advertise the drop-in to all pupils.

Being able to talk to a school about specific needs that are highlighted by pupils is a valuable tool for service delivery.

Drop-in work has become more common in schools across the UK. A range of health and social issues are seen by the school nurse on a one-to-one basis. School nurses are trusted adults who young people can access for advice and help, and the school nurse can develop a therapeutic relationship or can signpost young people on to other services if necessary. Understanding multi-professional working and utilising appropriate skills within the school health team is essential. School nurses must understand their role and maintain professional relationships to provide quality services. These issues are discussed further in Chapters 2 and 6.

School nurse-led services

Increasingly, school nurses are leading projects and interventions. Their role in leading immunisation teams in schools is well established having taken over this role from the school doctors. Campaigns such as the human papilloma virus vaccination programme fall within the remit of the school health service and impact significantly on stretched services. Across the country, enuresis clinics have become the domain of the school nurses and projects around weight management have also been established in some areas. In order to provide the services and continue with important projects, the issue of resources must be explored further. The Public Health white paper *Health Lives, Healthy People* (DH, 2010) outlined a key emphasis on young people, their education and their health. The school health service is also outlined within the paper, and although it is envisaged that teams will be of different levels and skills, it will still be the responsibility of school nurse team leaders to demonstrate the effectiveness of school health to the commissioners of services. It is important that commissioners recognise and fully understand the unique skills that the school nurse teams have to deliver public health services and the Healthy Child Programme (DH/DCSF, 2009). This is explored further in Chapter 7.

A day in the life of a school nurse

There follow two examples of newly-qualified school nurses as they begin their new roles. These two examples clearly demonstrate the diversity of the school nursing role and the fulfilling challenge that it presents.

A day in the life of a school nurse: Rachel Cabral

A wise lady once said to me: 'In this job you don't need to go looking for the work because it knows how to find you'.

It was a sunny September morning – my first day as a qualified school nurse – and as I drove to work I thought to myself how lucky I was. I had made it through the most challenging year of my life, the SCPHN course was over and now I could look forward to my new life as a school nurse.

I spent the first two days in my new office as any one would, getting to know the people and the paperwork and sorting out the mundane tasks, looking at a fairly empty diary: would I ever do any school nursing? Yet despite my anxiety to leap in and hunt for things to do, those words kept echoing in my mind.

Wise words well heeded indeed, for no sooner had I walked into the office on my third day than the phone rang. It had found me! An initial child protection conference. I sprang into action – I knew what I had to do, but the panic started to rise in my mind. I swathed through phone calls, visits and spent hours deliberating and writing the most comprehensive report I had ever written. I felt prepared and invincible, yet despite all the training and support I had received, I was totally unprepared for the emotional load it would place on me. I had been to several child protection conferences as a student, but this was different: my heart was pounding so loud it felt like the whole room could hear it. The lump in my throat was so big the words couldn't get past and those that did trembled. I came out of that meeting exhausted, thinking about the next phase of core group meetings.

Looking back now, it makes me smile to think about how nervous I felt. There are still times when I feel uncomfortable, but my confidence has grown and allows me to feel comfortable with my role in the process.

After that day, the work was true to form. It kept rolling in and the biggest lesson that I had yet to learn was how to say no. There haven't been two days the same. There is never a day where there is nothing to do, and some days I don't have time to stop and think. The variety in the job is truly marvellous: the days where the smallest thing feels like you have made a difference to someone's life are blended with the days where the world seems a cruel place. There are days when I have laughed and days where I have cried, but one thing keeps me going: knowing how important school nurses are to so many young people. My diary is full, days are filled weeks and months ahead. I have learned to plan my year ahead, arranging set sessions in the academic year prior. Drop-in sessions, immunisations, PSHE sessions, enuresis clinics, staff training and screening programmes are all planned well ahead so that there is some level of control in an ever-changing environment of work. With this control there is some relief from the uncertainty of child protection, and the day-to-day surprises that arise so regularly and need to be addressed. No two days are the same: there is no time to get bored. The diverse role of a school nurse is truly amazing.

A day in the life of a newly-qualified SCPHN: Liz Torres

8:45: I make my way across to the other side of the borough. At this point I'm feeling dreadfully guilty because I have just dropped my daughter off at school in a foul mood due to rushing. The dilemmas and guilt of being a working mum.

9:10: I find myself at my destination, outside a primary school. I have arranged to meet a dad to discuss his child's epilepsy and how this is managed at school. The school had been the primary source for the referral. They had originally requested training for rectal diazepam. Although there is nothing to say that schools cannot use rectal diazepam, buccal midazolam offers a more dignified mode of administration for the child involved, as well as maintaining the safety of both child and teachers in relation to safeguarding issues. All aspects of care have to be assessed and it is necessary to view care from all angles (child, parents and school), incorporating legal aspects such as policies (schools policies as well as our own nursing policies). Buccal midazolam should not be administered by school staff without previously receiving appropriate training, as this can affect their insurance policy. This is what I will be providing. However, it is first necessary to ensure that an individualised care plan is completed and that is the reason for the meeting I am having with the child's father.

I get a call from my colleague to inform me that the child's father is trying to contact me. I think to myself 'He wants to cancel' and 'What a waste of time this journey has been'. I call him and find out that he would rather meet up somewhere else. I agree and find him in a church hall coffee shop. I consider confidentiality issues, as there are other people present. I explain this to dad, but he has no concerns.

There is no medical needs pathway for school nursing in our borough; however, this is a role for the school nurse which is stipulated within our service level agreement. We follow recommendations from government. It is the responsibility of schools to ensure they have the appropriate policies, so I will discuss this with the school later.

After getting all the information I need to compile the care plan, I make a list of things to do: write care plan and nursing notes and place child on the computerised system; obtain consultant's signature, parent's signature and Head Teacher's signature on the care plan; book and deliver training to the school; and liaise with the GP to ensure the prescription is written in a way that will be clear to the pharmacist so that it is properly written on the label and comprehensible to the school staff.

10:30: From this meeting I make my way to the local secondary school where I deliver a 'Delay' session to a year 8 class. This is a session that offers young people strategies to delay early sexual activities. The session was planned in the last academic year whilst I was in supervised practice as a student. I thoroughly enjoy these sessions. All right: the thought of delivering sex education to a group of unruly teenagers can be a little daunting, but the key is to not show your fear and go with the flow. When things start getting out of hand, which inevitably they will because that is the whole nature of the topic, take a breath, smile and lower your voice by a couple of decibels. You'll soon see that they really do want to listen to what you have to say.

It's important to remember that they also want you to hear them, so make the session as interactive as possible, with a variety of teaching styles. I find that the most important points to get across are respect for themselves and keeping safe. Written evaluation forms are handed out just before the end of the session. A couple of these shock me. 'Name one thing you have learnt'... 'You can say no if you don't want sex'. At this point I think to myself PSHE and SRE are a vital part of a young person's education and the public health agenda, so why don't we do more?

11:30–12:30: I hold a school nursing open door session at the secondary school. This is held once a fortnight. Young people can access this service which offers confidential health-related information as necessary with no appointment needed. I eat a sandwich before I'm approached by a 14-year-old girl who is sexually active and has been sent to see me by the pastoral support teacher. I introduce myself and explain my role to her. I also explain that I am there to help her and the information she shares will be confidential and not shared with teachers or parents. I also explain that if I feel she is at significant risk then I will need to share that information with other agencies, but I will not do this without letting her know.

The girl tells me her story and I listen. Although it is not always possible to stick to open-ended questions, it is paramount that leading questions are not used. It is important to establish first and foremost if this girl is at risk of significant harm. Some questions that may be useful would be 'Tell me where you met him'; 'Is he your boyfriend?'; 'What year is he in?'. These types of questions enable you to assess if the girl is being taken advantage of without placing the idea of sexual abuse in her head. I establish that this young girl is Gillick-competent and is being responsible in seeking information. We explore issues such as feelings and drug and alcohol use. I offer her some sexual health advice and signpost her to the relevant sexual health clinic for further input. I remind her when I will be in school again and ask her to come and let me know how she gets on.

12:30: I go to the reception desk and look through the diphtheria, tetanus and polio consent forms. I obtain contact details to parents who have not given consent to immunisation and also those who have queries. It is important to establish the reason for non-consent, as explanation may aid compliance and hence improve uptake, which in turn will improve our statistics.

12:55: I'm at the doctor's surgery. I hope to talk to the GP regarding the care plan I started this morning. I wait outside her door and catch her as her previous patient leaves. We discuss the care plan and she writes a prescription to be delivered to the pharmacy for collection by the parents. She mentions that she didn't realise that there were still school nurses... ha ha. We have a little chat and I educate her in the school nursing role.

13:20: I'm at another primary school where I have arranged to meet the Head Teacher. She has contacted me to ask for advice on implementing a sex and relationship education policy. I have liaised with head teachers from two other primary schools to gain their consent to share their SRE policy – they were more than happy to help. I have also compiled a ring folder with the national and borough guidelines, the two model policies and an array of leaflets for young people relating to the topic. I have borrowed a selection of DVDs from the Health Promotion Resources Department and I have included a leaflet from this department which will aid the school in obtaining future resources for SRE as well as other health-related issues for PSHE.

I invite myself to a future School Governors Healthy Schools forum so that I can endorse (recommend) establishing the SRE policy. I also speak to the Head Teacher about the need for a good medical needs policy and explain that I would be happy to discuss this further at the forum. We discuss medical needs in her school and I establish that an epi-pen and asthma training update is necessary (I must remember to tell our staff nurse to book a session).

14:45: I return to the office feeling like I have not had a break all day. I make myself a cup of coffee, take a sip and check my messages. I have ten thousand things going through my head and realise that there are another ten thousand waiting for me. At least I have a couple of hours to focus on catching up with phone calls and paperwork. I find myself drawn into issues relating to colleagues and realise that another 30 minutes have passed trying to resolve these management issues.

Right! Focus! I take my cold cup of coffee into a separate office where I can channel my efforts into the various phone calls to social workers, schools, parents etc. I have to concentrate to prioritise my work effectively, otherwise I am easily distracted. What comes next? Sorting out the care plan that I have been doing this morning? Writing notes on the girl I saw at the open door? No. Although these are important, they can wait. I write a list in one of my three notebooks. This helps me prioritise and at least I won't forget anything. I cross items off my list as I go along, giving me a sense of achievement as the list grows unendingly longer (this is not a nonsensical error).

I've written in my diary to remind me of when things need to be done. I look at next week and see that I'm pretty organised (until other items crop up). Entries such as performing a child protection health assessment and allocating time to write a report for a CP conference are booked in. These I plan well in advance. However, I've not dealt with a health issue that arose at a core group so this will have to be resolved.

Reports take forever to write, but it does get easier, especially when having a caseload of 10 child protection families. I remember that I had composed a letter at home and emailed it to myself at work. This email explains to my manager that I am not happy to take on any further child protection cases, as I feel that my practice would become unsafe were I to do so. I copy in the Children's Services Manager and the Clinical Governance Lead. A weight has been lifted from my shoulders. I feel that if issues such as these are not highlighted, then we cannot move forward as a service. Commissioners need to be aware of such issues, and by doing this the ownership of the problem is passed on to them and my manager will have the ammunition necessary to use.

I enter the computerised system and log in my 'face-to-face contact' which is vital in demonstrating my activity (again, more ammunition). We have not yet entered into the RiO computerised system but this is approaching fast. I believe that if an organisation has made the effort to supply thousands of pounds worth of computers, printers and scanners, then they must be taking this seriously. We need to learn to use it to our advantage. Nowadays we cannot say we are too busy to do something – this needs to be quantified. Like I say: ammunition! Gone are the ward days where I would be sent to find something to do. Being busy is much more rewarding. I finish writing up nursing notes. I look through my list to make sure I have done what I can, whilst adding a couple more items to follow up tomorrow.

17:20: I feel like I could work for a couple more hours, but I decide to go home feeling I have done my bit for today. Tomorrow is another day and just as busy no doubt!

Conclusion

In conclusion, this book was written at a time of political change and unrest for health and social care services. The Health and Social Care Bill (DH, 2011) was stalled in 2011 for a 'listening exercise' when many pressure groups opposed its radical changes to the NHS. In January 2012, the Royal College of Nurses and the

Royal College of Midwives joined the British Medical Association and the Royal College of General Practitioners in outright opposition to the bill. Prime Minister David Cameron's vision of 'the big society' is underpinned by the Health and Social Care Bill and he insisted that the fundamental principles of the NHS would not change with the reforms. The commissioning agenda seems set to endure however, despite this opposition, and school nurses need to continue to be mindful of this in the pursuit of promoting the health and wellbeing of children, young people and their families using quality frameworks of care. The Health and Social Care Bill finally achieved Royal Assent on March 27th 2012.

References

BBC (2010) *The Do Gooders: Suffer the Little Children.* First broadcast BBC2, 6 December.

British Youth Council [BYC] (2011) *More That Just Jabs.* Available at: http://www.byc.org.uk/news/more-than-just-jabs-someone-to-trust.aspx (accessed 28 December 2011).

Change4life (2012) Available at: http://www.nhs.uk/change4life/Pages/change-for-life.aspx.

Chief Nursing Officer Bulletin (2011) *Profile: School Nurse (Jessica Streeting).* Available at: http://www.dh.gov.uk/en/Publicationsandstatistics/Bulletins/Chiefnursingofficerbulletin/September2011/DH_130030 (accessed 21 January 2012).

Department for Education [DfE] (2010) *The Importance of Teaching: the Schools White Paper.* DfE, London.

Department for Education (2011) *Academies.* Available at: http://www.education.gov.uk/schools/leadership/typesofschools/academies (accessed 26 January 2011).

Department of Health [DH] (2004a) *National Service Framework for Children, Young People and Maternity Services.* DH, London.

Department of Health (2004b) *Choosing Health: Making Healthy Choices Easier.* DH, London.

Department of Health (2010) *Healthy Lives, Healthy People.* DH, London.

Department of Health (2011) *The Health and Social Care Bill.* DH, London.

Department of Health (2012a) *Getting it Right for Children, Young People and Their Families. Maximising the Contribution of the School Nursing Team. Vision and Call to Action.* DH, London.

Department of Health (2012b) *Improving Outcomes and Improving Transparency. Part 1: A Public Health Outcomes Framework (2013–2016).* DH, London.

Department of Health/Department for Children, Schools and Families (2008) *Transition: Moving on Well.* DH/DCSF, London.

Department of Health/Department for Children, Schools and Families (2009) *The Healthy Child Programme from 5 to 19.* DH/DCSF, London.

Department of Health/Department for Education and Skills (2004) *Every Child Matters: Change for Children.* DH/DfES, London.

Hall, D. and Elliman, D. (eds) (2003) *Health for All Children*, 4th edn. Oxford University Press, Oxford.

Health and Safety Executive [HSE] (2009) *Working Alone; Health and Safety Guidance on the Risks of Working Alone.* HSE, London.

HM Government (2006) *Working Together to Safeguard Children.* Stationery Office, London.

Health Protection Agency [HPA] (2011) *Guidance on Infectious Diseases in Schools and Other Childcare Settings.* Available at: http://www.hpa.org.uk/web/ HPAweb&HPAwebStandard/HPAweb_C/1203496946639 (accessed 15 December 2011).

Multi-systemic Therapy [MST] (2011) Available at: http://www.nmhdu.org.uk/news/multi-systemic-therapy-new-therapy-brings-results-for-troubled-young-people/ (accessed 29 November 2011).

National Institute for Clinical Health and Excellence [NICE] (2003*) Infection Control.* Available at: http://guidance.nice.org.uk/CG2/Guidance/pdf/English (accessed 15 December 2011).

NICE (2007) *Prevention of Sexually Transmitted Infections and Under 18 Conceptions (PH3).* Available at: http://guidance.nice.org.uk/PH3 (accessed 21 January 2012).

Nightingale, F. (1860) *Notes on Nursing.* Harrison, London.

Nuffield Council on Bioethics (2007) *Public Health: Ethical Issues.* Nuffield Council on Bioethics, London.

Nursing and Midwifery Council [NMC] (2004) *Standards of Proficiency for SCPHN.* NMC, London.

Nursing and Midwifery Council (2006) *Preceptorship Guidelines.* NMC, London.

Nursing and Midwifery Council (2008) *The Code.* NMC, London.

Underwood, J. E. A. (1946) School health service in England and Wales. *American Journal of Public Health*, **36**(7), 703–10.

United Nations Development Programme (2012) *Empowered Lives, Resilient Nations.* Available at: http://www.beta.undp.org/undp/en/home.html.

Robothom, A. and Frost, M. (2005) *Health Visiting: Specialist Community Public Health Nursing.* Elsevier, London.

Wanless, D. (2004) *Securing Good Health for the Whole Population.* HM Treasury, London.

Wright, J. (2011) Public health history and the emergence of school nursing *British Journal of School Nursing*, **6**(6)

CHAPTER 2

Essential skills for school nurses

Sharon Aldridge-Bent and Jane Wright

Key themes in this chapter:

■ What personal skills do I need?
- Self-awareness
- Assertiveness
- Reflective skills
- Communication skills
■ What skills do I need to support and manage staff?
■ How do I keep up to date?
■ Teaching and learning in practice
■ What other key skills will I need?
- Knowledge of child development
- Planning care
- Record keeping
- Organisational skills

Introduction

There are fundamental skills that all school nurses will need in order to practise both safely and effectively. This chapter will explore some of those key skills, and although some are also discussed elsewhere, this chapter provides further supportive literature to underpin the knowledge.

What personal skills do I need?

The leadership role for school nurses is becoming ever more important. It is implicit throughout the Healthy Child Programme (DH/DCSF, 2009) and explicit in the service model for school nursing practice (DH, 2012). The qualities of a leader in dealing with difficult situations are explored further in Chapter 3, and in addition to those qualities there are personal skills such as self-awareness, assertiveness and reflection which enrich the role as a leader as well as a practitioner.

Self-awareness

When considering leadership and its purpose in the school nurse setting, it is important that as a leader you have a degree of self-awareness in terms of how you present yourself to others and how others perceive you (Tyler, 2004).

A common tool used to identify personal qualities is a SWOT analysis. This is a good way to establish insight into your own abilities. Take a sheet of paper and divide it into four cells and label them 'Strengths', 'Weaknesses', 'Opportunities' and 'Threats'. Under each heading within each cell, write down as many things that you can think of that relate to your role as a leader. You can then ask yourself 'What are the threats that the weaknesses expose us to?' and 'What opportunities arise because of your strengths?' (Tyler, 2004). Doing a SWOT analysis allows you to become critical and to reflect upon your own behaviour. This can sometimes be a step towards changing and developing both personally and professionally as a result of this self-analysis.

The SWOT analysis can also assist in identifying your own personal leadership style and also areas where you may be lacking. The true acceptance of your own limitations or shortcomings may ultimately be significant in being able to delegate to others.

> No one person could possibly stay on top of everything.... Only when leaders come to see themselves as incomplete, as having both strengths and weaknesses, will they be able to make up for their missing skills by relying on others (Ancona *et al.*, 2007, p. 94).

The need for delegation in school nursing has become more important as resources become stretched, and it is explicit in all guidance for school nursing practice (DH, 2012). Further discussion around delegation is contained in Chapter 5 in relation to Personal, Social, Health and Economic education. It is also explored further in Chapter 7 on needs assessment.

Assertiveness

Exploring self-awareness will almost certainly influence how a personal leadership style is developed. Your staff may look to you to lead the way, but this does not mean that you have to have all the answers, only that you can provide clarity of direction. To achieve this, there must be a certain amount of self-confidence and self-belief. Martin *et al.* (2010) argue that this will include how you 'carry yourself', your appearance, your voice, posture and manner.

You need to learn the art of acting, of appearing confident even if inside you are scared... most important is learning to be confident (Stewart, 1989, p. 11).

By establishing this personal authority, an inner confidence can emerge that can assist in influencing others. Being assertive is a way of influencing people, achieved through open, direct and honest communication. This communication is developed by valuing others, listening, respecting, problem solving and negotiating with other people. Being assertive means respecting yourself and other people, seeing people as equal to you, not better than you or less important than you. The goal of assertive behaviour is to stand up for your rights in such a way that you do not violate someone else's. Becoming more assertive does not mean that you always get what you want, but it can help you achieve a compromise. It is much easier to be assertive in situations where you are confident about your knowledge and skills base. Therefore, alongside developing communication skills, keeping up to date and reflecting on your practice are key skills.

Reflective skills (guided dialogue)

In all professional roles it is important to reflect upon a situation, whether it is deemed as positive or negative. Reflection is seen as a theory of critical thinking and is a process of reviewing an experience of practice in order to describe, analyse, evaluate and so inform learning about practice (Boud *et al.*, 1985). Invariably, it is human nature to reflect upon an occurrence when 'something has gone wrong' (Taylor and White, 2000). Reflective practice advocates that we should reflect upon good practice as a way of enhancing and reinforcing the practice as well as being a quality control mechanism.

There are many models of reflection that can be used to assist in reflection. Models may be viewed as academic exercises that at times are poorly implemented and poorly understood by practitioners (Quinn, 2008). However, the model that is used is not as important as long as a process occurs. Johns' (1992) model of reflection is commonly applied, the basics of which are:

- Experience
- Perception
- Making sense
- Principles
- Application

In exploring these, reflection becomes more than just thoughtful practice; it becomes a process of turning thoughtful practice into a potential learning situation

(Johns, 1992). The learning that occurs must be in some way utilised, and if it is viewed that practices or behaviours must be changed then how these changes occur need to be considered:

> Reflection without action is wishful thinking (Freire [1972] cited in Ghaye [2011])

Commonly, reflection occurs when there is a critical incident, and Wood (1998) identified a useful framework which guides practitioners to review practice and plan action:

1. Description of what took place during the incident.
2. Analysis of the situation, exploring the communication skills used and clarification of the underpinning moral values.
3. Exploration of potentially effective alternative strategies to those skills actually employed, including moral justification for proposed alternatives.
4. Identification of implications for practice.

As leaders, school nurses may also use these reflective models with members of staff when supporting them through critical incidents or clinical supervision. The key is to have a clear action plan following reflection.

Reflexivity

The follow-up from reflection is the theory of reflexivity: this phenomenon has been widely used within other professions and in particular, social work. A distinction needs to be made between reflection and reflexivity. Reflexivity takes reflection one step further by scrutinising and making 'problems' of issues that reflection may take for granted. By doing this, reflexivity suggests that the things we take for granted need to be challenged in order to change theory, practice or behaviours (Taylor and White, 2000). This means that our preconceived ideas about our established practices require deeper exploration, and this in turn stops us from developing ritualistic or 'shallow' practice. This has really been a crucial issue within many areas of healthcare practice, and school nursing is no exception. Making change and managing entrenched views and practices is discussed further in Chapter 3.

Communication skills

Negotiation

Negotiation may take many different forms and requires you to perform in various ways (Fisher and Ury, 2003). To be a successful negotiator requires practice and skill. In some instances it may mean that you have to argue a point in order to succeed, while in others it may mean having to compromise, where both parties may lose something. The skills developed over time are related to bargaining skills and fall into two categories: principled bargaining and positional bargaining (Gates, 2011). Principled bargaining is where both parties work together and jointly analyse a problem to reach an agreed goal. It is meant to be more satisfying and fulfilling for both parties. Positional bargaining is based more on a bargaining technique where both parties come with a set ideas of what the outcome should be; it invariably ends up with one or both parties having to be more tactical in order to win the other over (Fisher and Ury, 2003). The skill is to be able to recall which strategy you are using in which circumstances, or to be able to skilfully switch from one to the other in order to achieve your own goal.

Fletcher (1998) in Parahoo (2006) suggests that successful negotiation is about four things:

- Being clear what you want
- Understanding the context
- Preparing the ground
- Managing yourself and coping with the encounter

A key point to remember here is to consider the person or group you are negotiating with. At the heart of school nursing practice are the needs of children and young people, and this must be at the forefront of negotiations.

Examples of negotiations

- With a parent about a child's health needs
- With a young person about, for example: smoking cessation, their sexual activity, non-attendance at school or their alcohol intake
- With a school, head teacher or governors about an initiative that you have identified as important within your needs assessment (for example, a health drop-in – see Chapter 6)
- With managers or commissioners around resource issues
- With a GP about sharing information
- With other agencies about a particular child or young person's need

With these examples, you can identify which negotiation techniques may be used (principled or positional) and remember that the fundamental role of the school nurse is to act in the best interests of children and young people, which may require tough negotiation skills.

Conflict resolution

Not all negotiation will end positively, and you may need to resolve a conflict. Conflict resolution requires time to discuss and explore problems in order for it to be performed well, and it should be a priority (Ramsbottom *et al.*, 2011). Within the school nurse setting, protected time or an appropriate environment needs to be promoted to allow for issues to be resolved. Traditionally, within nursing it has been acknowledged that nurses do not always feel that they are equipped to deal with conflict (Ramsbottom *et al.*, 2011). This view is changing somewhat with the emergence of new leadership roles within the profession, and in particular in school nursing.

Managing conflict can present as a challenge and there are many examples of the need to use these skills: for example, dealing with angry parents at child protection conferences or following school nurse input without parental knowledge. The key here is to be fully cognisant of the local protocols and procedures that are in place as well as the law (see Fraser guidelines in Chapter 6) and the NMC guidelines (NMC, 2008a). School nurses can then talk to parents confidently in the knowledge that they have acted in the best interests of the child or young person within their range of expertise and job description. This way, they cannot be accused of acting negligently. An issue may arise if the anger is aimed at a member of your team, and you will need to deal with this promptly (see Chapter 3).

General tips about resolving conflict

- Do not match the other person's anger. Speak calmly, do not raise your voice and allow them to air their views. Often the anger will subside if you allow them space to talk.
- Be safe; make sure that if anger does not subside quickly that you rearrange a time for them to calm down and for you to have someone with you.
- Be clear that you will not tolerate abuse and neither will the organisation that you work for.
- Actively listen to what they are saying and acknowledge their views using appropriate eye contact, open body language and clarification techniques so that you are absolutely clear about what the problem is.
- Make notes and if necessary tell the other party that you are going to do so.
- Before responding, make sure you do not say anything which may incriminate you. You might want to make another meeting to give you time to think, investigate or get advice.
- If possible, you can respond by explaining your actions or the actions of others in your team in a calm, considered way and be clear about what protocols or procedures that you have followed.

See Activity 2.1 for an activity on negotiation skills.

Activity 2.1 Resolving conflict

Think about a situation you have been in where you have had to negotiate with an individual to resolve a conflict. List answers to the following questions:

- How clear were you about what you wanted?
- How did you relay this to the individual?
- How did you present yourself?
- When negotiating in the future are there any changes you would implement as a result of this experience?

Facilitating skills

It takes a skilled and well-prepared facilitator to ensure that groups work effectively. School nurses may be required to facilitate groups of children and young people, parents, students or colleagues. There will be a number of reasons why you may need to facilitate groups, but generally speaking you are either assessing the knowledge level of a group or generating information (for example if you are creating a protocol).

The facilitator needs to be able to do the following:

1. Be directive when organising the group, e.g. allocate people into groups as opposed to allowing people to form their own. This technique works on two levels: firstly it randomly selects the group members so that there are diverse opinions within the group and people have not selected each other based on 'like mindedness'. In a classroom situation, this is very helpful to avoid disruptive groups forming. Secondly, it assists in swiftly organising group participation, which otherwise can be time-consuming as people try to self-select, or are unable to self-select if they do not know each other.

2. Once the groups have finally settled, explain what is required of them and check that everyone understands. Also, establish how long you want them to work on the exercise for and what the expectation is from them at the end. What information are you trying to establish?

3. A good group facilitator then allows the group to get on with the task at hand without any interruptions. At no stage should the facilitator join the group unless group members invite them for clarity of the task. The facilitator

should only assist with a specific need and then remove themselves from the group. This allows the group to explore their own thoughts and ideas without the influence of the facilitator.

4. The facilitator should then manage the feedback session so that all participants feel that they have been given the opportunity to contribute equally.

5. Finally the facilitator should always thank the groups for their input and participation.

Further discussion on teaching young people in PSHE sessions is contained in Chapter 5.

Chairing meetings

Successful meetings are usually dependent on how they are facilitated and chaired (Yoder-Wise, 2011). In order for a meeting to be both fulfilling and productive with clear outcomes there are some key skills that should be developed by the chairperson.

If you have been identified as the Chair then do not be afraid to speak out and chair the meeting as you have been delegated to do. Some characteristics of a good Chair are to be directional, have good listening and analytical skills and be inclusive (Peberdy and Hammersley, 2009). It is also important as the Chair that all participants feel that they have been listened to. Never see a meeting as an opportunity to get your own views across or attempt to dominate the discussion if you are chairing the meeting (Peberdy and Hammersley, 2009). By the same token, as the Chair, try to discourage private or irrelevant conversations politely as the group can drift off-topic very quickly.

It is good practice to have a written agenda for all meetings. This is simply a list of all the things that you wish to discuss. It assists in keeping the meeting focused and structured upon the intended topic. It is also useful to have rough timings for how long each item may take to discuss and be realistic about how long things may take to resolve. Don't be tempted to put too much into the agenda: discussions will invariably take longer than you think.

As the Chair it is important to have a clear idea of the length of the meeting, as it is not recommended that a meeting be longer than two hours if you want it to be productive (Peberdy and Hammersley, 2009). The running of a meeting may vary depending upon the type of meeting, and this needs to be communicated by the Chair from the outset. An opening statement and explanation of the general direction and rules of the meeting may help to eliminate any issues that may occur later – for example, interruptions, adherence to the agenda and the need for certain decisions to be made. It will also be necessary to establish that discriminatory language or behaviour will not be tolerated. It is always good practice to have a minute taker and for any action points agreed to be clearly identified and the people responsible for the actions to be noted. It is difficult to do this as the Chair. Finally, a good Chair should be able to recap and summarise the salient points and bring the meeting to an appropriate close, ensuring that all parties are aware of their responsibilities, time frames for action points and times of next meetings.

There is a real skill to moving a meeting forward and sometimes it is difficult to 'contain' very vocal members of groups. There is a balance between allowing people to have their say and allowing them to dominate the meeting. As a Chair, you need to be respectful but assertive about moving discussions on.

General tips for chairing meetings

- Start on time; don't be tempted to wait for members to arrive, as time is precious in practice.
- Start with introductions unless you are sure everyone knows each other, but keep this as short as possible.
- Opening statement about the purpose of the meeting and how long you anticipate it will last.
- Stick closely to the agenda and keep people on task.
- Make sure that you are actively listening to what people are saying, and show respect.
- Challenge any discriminatory language or behaviour.
- Be assertive: allow people to have their say, but stop them if the discussion is irrelevant or drifts off-topic. You can use phrases like '...that is interesting, but it is a discussion for another time...' or '..thank you for your input, that's really helpful, we now need to move on...'. Holding up your hand to show someone that they have had their time is useful.
- Allocate any actions to specific people. Be wary of taking on everything yourself; delegate to others if possible.
- Ensure that you have a closing round to give those who have not contributed much a chance to speak. Allow some time at the end for this.
- Recap on what people are expected to do for the next meeting.
- Make dates and times for the next meeting.

Listening and communicating with young people

School nurses are not counsellors, although some will have some training in this area. However, they use counselling skills every day in order to communicate and listen to children, young people, parents, colleagues and others. School nurses have to make judgements about what is required in different situations dependent on who they are talking to. Some individuals will be wanting specific health advice, some will have specific mental health problems and others will be seeking a 'listening ear'. There is a skill in recognising the differences between these situations, and listening in the first instance is the key. There are some considerations when talking to children and young people on an individual basis:

- **Consider position**: This needs to be comfortable for you and the young person. This may mean sitting to one side rather than directly in front. Avoid a barrier between you, such as a desk or table.
- **Body language**: You should be relaxed and open. Sitting forward slightly tends to demonstrate attentiveness. Crossed arms can be seen as defensive. You can also take the opportunity to observe the young person's body language. Are they agitated, worried, uncomfortable, restless, constantly looking at the door, reluctant to engage? These may mean that they are not really ready to talk to you or that they are nervous and may take time to settle down. As nurses we also make an assessment of their physical appearance – are they tired, pale, thin, overweight? – etc.
- **Eye contact**: Be careful with eye contact. It is good to show that you are interested in the young person, but they can find it threatening if you stare. In some cultures, eye contact is seen as disrespectful, so judge each situation on its own merit.
- **Privacy**: Ensure that you have no interruptions when talking on a one-to-one basis. Turn off your phone and ensure that no one is going to disturb you for the duration of the session.
- **Listen carefully**: Active listening means that you need to ensure that you understand what is being said. This can be problematic with adolescents when they use language that you may not understand. Feed back and clarify as you go along, but don't interrupt. Don't be tempted to fill silences: wait for the young person to speak and give them time to do so.
- **Be non-judgemental**: You may not like what the young person is telling you, but in order to build trust, you must remain neutral in your expressions and body language. However, you must follow guidelines on confidentiality and child protection.
- **Show empathy**: No one can fully understand another person's experience, as this is unique to them, but you can show that you are sensitive to their situation.
- **Confidentiality**: You must establish from the start that you may have to disclose information to others if you are worried about the young person's safety.

■ **Consider clear 'endings'**: Agree timings and keep to time for the sessions. Young people will respond better to a structure. They will begin to trust you if you do as you say you are going to do. Equally, agree how many times you need to talk and fix that at the first session if necessary.

Tools and resources to consider when engaging young people

The key to working with children and young people is to recognise your own limitations. It is very important to work within your range of expertise and capabilities and this relates back to being self aware. It is also about being aware of referral routes and care pathways to ensure that if you feel that young people need more help, that you know where to signpost them to. Working with other agencies will also protect you and make you feel more secure and confident about the work that you are doing. However, it is useful to consider some of the common approaches and strategies that are used to engage young people.

■ **Client-centred approaches**: As the name suggests these approaches put the client at the centre of any intervention and are a non-directive approach to counselling. It refers to the notion that any changes to behaviour must be generated from the client (or young person) and that the role of the 'therapist' is to facilitate that change. Carl Rogers (1953) is perhaps one of the most quoted authors on client-centred therapy and his book *Client-Centred Therapy* is a useful resource.

■ **Solution-focused work**: Rather than concentrating on problems, it is felt that, ideally, one should be helping individuals to move forward positively away from the problems in their lives. This does not mean that you do not talk about the problems, as clearly they will have to be explained, but it is about finding out how people can identify what they want to do about those problems. This can often be extremely difficult with children and young people, who may feel they have no control over the circumstance in which they live. Small steps are important – this gives more control to young people. If they can solve the smaller problems in their lives, they will begin to feel more confident that they can succeed with the bigger ones. Feeling in control of our lives is crucial to our self-esteem and a loss of control can lead to being bullied (see Chapter 3). Setting objectives for the next time you meet is useful, but keep these objectives achievable and realistic.

■ **Art and imagery**: This can be either guided or not. 'Free' art is used often to allow children and young people to express their feelings as they wish. This can be very powerful (Case study 2.1). School nurses should be wary, however, of interpreting artwork and reaching inappropriate conclusions unless they have been specifically trained in this area. Asking individuals to draw pictures about their lives and what the future holds can be useful too. For example, thinking about life as a road with many turnings can help them to think about what may influence them to take a wrong turning, what they could do to prevent that happening and what happens when they come to a crossroads. Young children can be asked to draw a house with all the people in their family in it. You can then build a picture about how the child is feeling about their lives. Story books can also be used with young children, either to help illustrate that problems are not unique to them, as in *The Huge Bag of Worries* by Virginia Ironside (2004), but also as talking points. School nurses can build up a stock of resources such as books, play-dough, Lego, paper and crayons that are easily transportable.

Case study 2.1

Sophie was 15 and attended a high-achieving girls' grammar school. She came to the school nurse drop-in at lunchtime one day because she was self-harming and was very troubled about her life and future. The school nurse listened carefully to Sophie's story, which pivoted on a very unhappy family where her father had died when she was 10 and her mother had remarried and had two more children. In the first session, the school nurse simply listened to Sophie and allowed her some time to talk. After that, Sophie came regularly and it was clear that her self-harming behaviour was very serious. Sophie would show the school nurse her injuries and she had been admitted to hospital on several occasions. She had been referred to the GP and Child and Adolescent Mental Health services by both the hospital and the school nurse, but the referral was taking time to be processed.

The story of her family life became gradually more alarming as the weeks went by and it was clear that Sophie needed more help than the school nurse alone could give. Sophie had been sexually abused by her father. Her mother had not believed her and had remarried a man who also went on to abuse Sophie, and her mother did not believe her then either. In fact, her mother accused Sophie of making up stories, because how could two men that she had married possibly do that? A child protection plan was in place and the stepfather left the family home, causing more resentment from the mother.

The school nurse worked closely with CAMHS, who were professionally treating Sophie for very complex psychological problems. CAMHS were also helping mum to listen to Sophie. However, Sophie had developed a trusting relationship with the school nurse and liked coming to see her, not just to talk but also to draw and paint. The school nurse allowed her to just come and sit and draw and paint for half an hour a week for six months. Sometimes she would talk about what she was drawing, sometimes not. Sophie said that this space for her in the school each week allowed her quiet thinking time, which meant that she could focus better on her school work, and also had a calming effect on her, which reduced the cutting behaviour significantly. It also allowed her to talk more to her mum about the situation. This demonstrates a good multi-agency approach, but also that – sometimes – young people need time and space which is just for them, with no pressure to talk.

- **Play**: Play therapy is a specialised therapeutic intervention, but school nurses can use play to help children talk or demonstrate how they are feeling in an informal way. Care must be taken of course to gain parental consent for any work with young children, and school nurses also need to be wary of using 'leading questions'. As with artwork, unless specifically trained, school nurses should be careful about interpreting the play. This should be an opportunity for listening and forming a relationship with young children. Any concerns raised in these sessions should be shared with appropriate people.

- **Protective behaviours**: school nurses in some areas are involved in delivering protective behaviours programmes. The programme focuses on two key themes: 'We all have the right to feel safe all of the time' and 'We can talk with someone about anything even if it is awful or small'. It can be useful in groups and on an individual basis to allow people to explore their feelings, identify early warning signs that something is wrong and explore supportive networks that can help. Although the programme is based on an anti-abuse idea, some of the strategies can be used on a more general level to help children and young people to talk – in particular, the network building and reviewing strategy. There is an initial identification of a trusted network of adults, which can be done by drawing around your hand and naming people in each of the fingers and the palm. A flower is sometimes used, with the names of people written in the petals. This can be kept and reviewed periodically and added to if you are seeing the young person on a number of occasions. It is really useful to do this because it prevents young people becoming dependent on you. It is much better that they build up a network that they can trust to talk to when you are no longer available. More information on the protective behaviours programmes can be found at http://www.protectivebehaviours.co.uk/.

- **Coaching and mentoring**: These terms are used to describe a supportive relationship that enables people to make their own decisions. The terms are used in many different areas of life, but for young people it is about the encouragement and support that they need to make decisions on a range of issues to help them in the future. Coaching implies training, and as young people move into adulthood, it could be argued that this is a crucial time for them to learn life skills, and looking after their own health and wellbeing is a life skill. School nurses have a role to play in providing good information for young people about their physical and mental health and to be clear about any risks they be taking. Mentoring implies giving support and advice as someone learns and grows in confidence. The ideal mentor is one who knows when to let the person go and allow them to move on without them. This is crucial for school nurses: they must not allow an interdependency to develop where both parties find it hard to let go. This can be likened to the parent/child relationship: a healthy relationship allows the child to become independent within a supportive and loving environment.

- **Motivational interviewing**: Motivational interviewing as a technique has arisen since the 1980s, and unlike the client-centred approach proposed by Carl Rogers, there is an element of direction in it. It was first used with problem drinkers to understand their behaviour and lack of motivation to change, but it may have a place in talking to young people. It is based on four general principles:

1. **Express empathy**
2. **Develop discrepancy**: This means examining where young people are in their lives and where they would like to be in the future. This is useful for exploring with young people about where they see themselves after leaving school. You can then explore how they think their behaviour may affect that future goal. Of course, there may be difficulties with young people who see no future for themselves, and this may require specialist help.
3. **'Roll with resistance'**: This means not fighting or challenging any resistance that young people may have to change but trying to understand it from their perspective. In terms of young people, this can be very effective because they may have been experiencing a strong, negative reaction from other adults about their behaviour and showing them that you are not judging the decision they are making will help them trust you.

4. **Supporting self-efficacy**: This relates to autonomy and how much control over change the young person has. It is also about respecting the choice that the young person makes, even if you feel it is the wrong decision. Showing that you understand that young people have a right to make choices in life helps to develop trust. Of course, this must lie within a safeguarding framework and any risks of significant harm must be acted upon.

- **Choices and consequences**: School nurses may be asked to help with the behaviour of young people that is directly impacting on others – for example, children or young people with anger management problems, bullies, or those with specific conditions such as ADHD. An assessment in these cases is needed, as are referrals on to other agencies if necessary. Good, established pathways of care are useful. Understanding the behaviour is very important, and this involves the listening and observational skills of school nurses to really understand what is happening. School nurses may be able to work through specific programmes with these children and young people, and considering choices and consequences of actions may be useful. With every choice that is made there is a consequence (for every action there is a reaction). Scenarios may be used in order to distance the discussion from the first person, and questions like 'What do you think will happen if this child hits another child?' may be similarly helpful. Stories may be useful with young children. Action plans should be agreed with the child or young person so that they are clear about what they have to do if, for example, they become angry. This will need to be agreed with others, such as the school, teachers, learning support assistants and educational psychologists, depending on the severity of the behaviour. Essentially, the children need to be able to remove themselves from the situation, talk to a trusted adult and understand why they are behaving in this way.

What skills do I need to support and manage staff ?

Part of the role of a manager is to develop the effective performance of staff members. Good practice is to take a structured approach to training and development of staff, including needs analysis and the development of a training plan and reviewing process. Managing a team that may have a diverse composition requires considerable skills. If you only consider people as individuals you could run the risk of ignoring some of the powerful influences that determine how effectively a team works (Walshe and Smith, 2011); these are discussed further in Chapter 3.

When managing others it is important to help people to flourish. This may involve enabling and challenging them. If you are not supporting, enabling and challenging then you are not managing. It takes this combination to assist people to realise their potential, and three basic rules for managing people are:

- Agree what is expected to be achieved.
- Be confident that they have the skills and resources to be able to achieve.
- Give constructive ongoing feedback about whether or not they are achieving.

These principles are explicit within the Knowledge and Skills Framework (KSF) produced alongside *Agenda for Change* in 2004. Agenda for Change was the review of the all-NHS pay and conditions of service:

> Staff are placed in one of nine pay bands on the basis of their knowledge, responsibility, skills and effort needed for the job. The assessment of each post, using the Job Evaluation Scheme (JES), determines the correct pay band for each post, and as a result, the correct basic pay. Within each pay band, there are a number of pay points. As staff successfully develop their skills and knowledge, they progress in annual increments up to the maximum of their pay band, At two defined 'gateway points' on each pay band, pay progression is based on them demonstrating the applied knowledge and skills for that job (Agenda for Change, 2012).

The KSF, in theory, was introduced to support staff in their career progression through personal and professional development. The key aims of the KSF are to help staff:

- Have clear and consistent development objectives.
- To develop in such a way that they can apply the knowledge and skills appropriate to their level of responsibility.
- To identify and develop knowledge and skills that will support their career progression.

New guidance on the KSF was issued in 2010 following a review to clarify and simplify the use of the KSF and emphasise that it can be adapted to local needs. The document provides useful templates for use in appraisals (KSF Guidelines, 2010). There is recognition within this guide that no 'one process' will fit with the many different structures within the NHS, and therefore the KSF is a framework on which to build healthy management processes locally.

There are six core dimensions within the KSF to be considered when forming local appraisal plans (KSF Guidelines, 2010, pp. 30–31):

- **Communication**: 'Communication has many forms and is a two-way process. It involves identifying what others are communicating as well as communicating yourself and the development of effective relationships'.
- **Personal and people development**: 'This dimension is about developing yourself and contributing to the development of others through both formal structured and informal *ad hoc* methods'.
- **Health, safety and security**: 'This dimension focuses on maintaining the health, safety and security of everyone in the organisation and anyone who comes into contact with it. It includes tasks that are undertaken as a routine part of work, such as moving or handling'.
- **Service improvement**: 'This dimension is about improving services in the interests of the users of those services and the public as a whole. The services might be services for the public (patients, clients and carers) or be services that support the smooth running of the organisation (such as finance, estates). The services might be single or multi-agency and uni- or multi-professional'.
- **Quality**: 'This dimension relates to maintaining high quality in all areas of work and practice, including the important aspects of effective team working. Quality can be supported using a range of different approaches including: codes of conduct and practice, evidence-based practice, guidelines, legislation, protocols, procedures, policies, standards and systems'.
- **Equality and diversity**: 'It is the responsibility of every person to act in ways that support equality and diversity. Equality and diversity [are] related to the actions and responsibilities of everyone – users of services including patients, clients and carers; work colleagues; employees, people in other organisations; the public in general'.

Within organisations, measuring performance is inherently linked to a business plan. 'People' form a major part of the resources needed to deliver a service, and a good business plan will include mechanisms for monitoring and measuring the effectiveness of those resources (see Chapter 7) (Walshe and Smith, 2011). Staff who perform poorly will impact on the overall cost effectiveness of the service delivery and this is crucial in a time of economic restraint. Appraisals are the process for not only identifying personal and professional development but also obtaining, analysing, and recording information about the relative worth of an employee within an organisation. They are a way of assessing an employee's recent successes and failures, personal strengths and weaknesses, and suitability for specific training, promotion or further performance management in some instances. The intention should be to support employees to improve their performance for the benefit of the whole service.

In most organisations, formal appraisals will be performed annually and then linked to personal and professional development plans for the coming year. They are formal written documents and are vital for managing the performance of people within an organisation. Performance appraisals should be positive experiences which provide a platform for development and motivation. Therefore organisations should foster a feeling that performance appraisals are positive opportunities for staff to develop and identify their needs.

Formal appraisals should include:

- Exploration of the previous year's objectives: have they been met and how?
- Consideration of less successful or less enjoyable elements of the role and exploration of why they are less enjoyable.
- Discussion on how performance is matching expectations. Do the knowledge and skills match the core dimensions of the KSF, or other occupational expectations or standards?
- The planning of objectives/goals for the coming year.
- Identification of any training needs to develop knowledge and skills in order to achieve the objectives.

However, waiting for a formal appraisal annually is not the best way to manage staff performance. Holding regular informal review meetings greatly reduces the pressure and time required for the annual formal appraisal meeting. In some organisations these monthly meetings are in the format of clinical supervision. The NHS Executive (1993) defines clinical supervision as a way of developing skills and knowledge in order to improve care. Clinical supervision enables registered nurses to:

- Identify solutions to problems
- Increase understanding of professional issues
- Improve standards of patient care
- Further develop their skills and knowledge
- Enhance their understanding of their own practice

The NMC supports the principle of clinical supervision but believes that it is best developed at a local level in accordance with local needs. It is perhaps for this reason that in some areas clinical supervision is well established and in others it does not have a high priority. School nurses will also have to consider staff members in their team who are not qualified nurses. Regular support and recognition of training needs will be important to maintain morale and ensure optimum levels of efficiency.

Preceptorship

The NMC strongly recommends that all 'new registrants' have a period of preceptorship on commencing employment NMC (2008b). Once a school nurse has completed the SCPHN programme, they will be a new registrant on the third part of the Register and it is acknowledged that this transition to an accountable practitioner requires support.

The role of the 'preceptor' is to:

- Facilitate and support the transition of a new registrant
- Facilitate the application of new knowledge and skills
- Raise awareness of the standards and competencies set that the new registrant is required to achieve and support to achieve these
- Provide constructive feedback on performance

Students finishing their SCPHN degree courses should have a preceptor for the first year of practice and they need to take some responsibility to ensure that this happens. This is a crucial area of support as part of their ongoing professional and personal development. The first year in practice is often a stressful time. The learning that has occurred at university in order to develop a deep level of knowledge and proficient skills in public health practice produces highly-motivated and professional individuals. The real nature of practice, with all its resource issues and other frustrations, can lead newly-qualified school nurses to become demoralised very quickly. A good preceptor will support the consolidation of knowledge and skills, be a listening ear and be positive in their approach to ensure that there is a low attrition rate among qualified school nurses.

How do I keep up to date?

In school nursing, as with other disciplines, keeping up to date is a requirement of the NMC registration. You are required to maintain currency in your field of practice to ensure that the best, evidence-based practice is maintained and therefore that the public is protected (NMC, 2011a). It is also crucial given the rapidly changing NHS that all nurses monitor changing policy and respond appropriately. Qualified SCPHNs are equipped with knowledge and skills from the degree courses that they undertake, but it is important that this is maintained throughout their careers.

One method of keeping updated is to perform a literature search (Table 2.1) of a particular topic of interest related to your practice. This is a way of broadening knowledge on a topic and it can increase both general and specialist knowledge. It facilitates a way of honing the skills of searching relevant material and allows

Table 2.1 The purpose of a literature search.

1. It broadens your knowledge on a topic.

2. Increases your general knowledge, specialist knowledge, vocabulary and confidence.

3. Shows your skill in finding relevant information.

4. Allows for critical appraisal of research.

for critical appraisal of research. It can also assist with developing an authority on a subject which contributes to being assertive when negotiating for resources (Gray, 2004).

A literature review is defined as a method for systematically identifying a body of completed and recorded work that has been produced by scholars, researchers and practitioners (Fink, 2005). It provides a rationale for decisions made and is used to answer a well-focused question or hypothesis about clinical practice (Cronin *et al.*, 2008). There are various reasons for searching the literature, such as to test a hypothesis, to answer a research question or simply to investigate a topic. This will in turn add to the body of knowledge that the nurse already has about the chosen topic. Once the literature has been identified it will be down to the researcher to decide how this information might be disseminated. In some instances the search may be performed to underpin a proposal for a larger or more in-depth piece of work or study. It may also be used to support a bid for resources.

The emerging themes and findings from a literature search can assist in raising both political and professional awareness and may identify gaps in evidence that would benefit from further exploration (Aveyard, 2010).

Contributing to consultation documents should also be an important aspect of the school nurse role. This means signing up to relevant professional forums such as the RCN or CPHVA school nurse forums and ensuring that you are on relevant email lists. Your managers will be on circulation lists from different organisations, such as government departments. Make sure that anything that is of interest is forwarded to you. Anyone can contribute to policy consultation documents, either as individuals or as groups, and this is crucial in raising the profile of school nurses. The consultation on school nursing led by the Department of Health in 2011 is testament to this because information was sent to all stakeholders across England, and organisations such as Mumsnet, the British Youth Council (BYC) and the National Children's Bureau (NCB) were consulted, providing solid evidence of the need for school nurses.

Teaching and learning in practice

Teaching and learning form a major part of the role of the school nurse from many perspectives. For much of their time, school nurses are involved in teaching or learning through their interactions with a wide range of individuals, including children, young people, parents, carers, colleagues, multidisciplinary team members and students. Teaching and learning are a two-way interaction, and one could argue that all experiences for the school nurse involve them either learning something themselves or teaching others. There is also a formal requirement for nurses to teach learners in practice, and a key mechanism for facilitating this is the mentoring system (Gopee, 2011). Mentorship of all learners is widely implemented and utilised both for pre- and post-registration nurses. As well as being a mentor, school nurses may want to become practice teachers as part of their continuing professional development.

The NMC (2008b) *Standards to Support Learning and Assessment in Practice* set out benchmarks and outcomes for mentors, practice teachers and teachers of midwives, nurses and SCPHNs. The standards identify a clear framework for the development of nurse teachers in four key stages:

- **Stage 1 NMC registrant**: reflects that all nurses and midwives must meet the defined requirements, in particular 'You must facilitate students and others to develop their competence' (NMC, 2008a).
- **Stage 2 Mentor**: nurses and midwives can become mentors when they have successfully achieved all the outcomes of this stage. This qualification is recorded on the local registers for mentors.
- **Stage 3 Practice teacher**: identifies the standard for a practice teacher for nursing or specialist community public health nursing. To become a practice teacher further outcomes need to be achieved. This qualification is recorded on a local register of practice teachers.
- **Stage 4 Teacher**: becoming a teacher upon successful completion of an NMC-approved programme when all outcomes for this stage have been achieved. This qualification is recorded on the NMC register.

There are five principles that underpin the above framework and dictate that the mentor/assessor must:

- Be on the same part of the register as that which the student is working towards.
- Have developed their knowledge and skills beyond registration.
- Hold a professional qualification equal to or at a higher level than that which the students are working towards.
- Have been prepared for their role and met the NMC outcomes for such.
- Record any NMC-approved teaching qualification on the register.

There are eight domains in the framework, which give guidance for applying the underpinning principles and have been designed for application within the context of interprofessional learning and working in modern healthcare (NMC, 2008b).

The eight developmental domains are:

- Establishing effective working relationships
- Facilitation of learning
- Assessment and accountability
- Evaluation of learning
- Creating an environment for learning
- Context of practice
- Evidence-based practice
- Leadership

See Activity 2.2 for an activity on teaching and learning.

Activity 2.2 Considering your learning environment

Think about your own practice area in relation to these eight domains and whether it is a healthy learning environment for all learners.

- Do you support learning with close links to your education services?
- Consider your relationship with your education provider.
- Do you know who your link tutor is?
- Do you have regular communication?
- What form does this communication take?
- How could the relationship be improved upon?

Responsibilities for teaching and learning of all members of the team

Team leader

The role of the team leader cannot be underestimated within the learning environment of the clinical setting. In order for learning to be achieved the team leader has to have a commitment to teaching and learning and have the ability to promote an atmosphere that encourages learning (Ogier, 1989). The facilitation of learning cannot be divorced from humane leadership and competent management. All areas of school nursing practice are potential learning environments that should foster and encourage learners of all kinds.

Community practice teacher

All SCPHN students must have a named practice teacher (NMC, 2008b). The role of the practice teacher is complex and requires an understanding of specialist practice. In order to be deemed a qualified practice teacher, an NMC-approved practice teacher programme needs to be undertaken. Practice teacher preparation programmes include at least 30 days protected learning time during which a trainee supports a student under the supervision of a sign-off practice teacher. Practice teachers are responsible and accountable for organising and coordinating the student's learning opportunities, assessing total performance and signing off achievement of proficiency.

In 2011, the NMC (2011b) gave additional guidance on supporting learning in practice. It outlined models for supporting more than one student at a time to facilitate a growing number of nurses being trained in specialist practice, particularly in health visiting. This raised concerns about the application of the NMC *Standards to Support Learning and Assessment in Practice* (NMC, 2008a). It was felt that student learning could be compromised as a result of these guidelines, and it is therefore crucial that local educational governance processes and policies are robust and transparent in order to ensure a safe educational environment (NMC, 2011b).

Being a practice teacher is a valuable and rewarding role for school nurses. It gives the opportunity to support learners, to be challenged on and (in practice) share their experiences, and to keep up to date. It is often a natural progression after a period of consolidation in practice. Many students return two or three years after qualifying to do the practice teacher course, despite having said they would never study again.

Mentor

According to the NMC, mentorship is 'a mandatory requirement for pre-registration nursing and midwifery students' (NMC, 2008b, p. 19). Mentors are accountable to the NMC for their decision that students are fit for practice and that they have the necessary knowledge, skills and competence to take on the role of registered nurse or midwife.

The NMC standard defines a mentor as being a registrant who has successfully completed an accredited mentor preparation programme from an approved Higher Education Institution. Pre-qualifying nurses (PQN) are increasingly being placed with school nurse teams, which should be viewed as a very positive development. Gaining insight into this very specialised public health role early on can inspire student nurses to go into school nursing after qualification. The view that nurses should work in a hospital before coming out into the community is an increasingly old-fashioned one. Community nurses (district nurses, health visitors, community children's nurses and school nurses) are specialists in their own right and should embrace newly-qualified nurses as the future community workforce. This is particularly poignant given the drive in recent years to care for people in the community rather than in the hospital setting. There are developing models across the country for students to do a four-year course, going straight on to SCPHN programmes direct from qualification after the three-year course.

Associate mentor

'Associate mentor' is the term given to an unqualified mentor who may be looking after a learner in the absence of the main mentor. In an area where there are many students and fewer qualified mentors this is educationally good practice. It also allows the learner to observe different ways of working and to witness a wider range of skills (Walsh, 2010).

Learner

'Learner' is the term given to any person who has identified learning outcomes that may need to be achieved within the clinical setting. The person could be a PQN, a qualified nurse doing a continuing professional course, a healthcare assistant or a nurse who is new to the area of practice. The development of skill mix in school nursing leads to qualified school nurses increasingly teaching new members of staff: community staff nurses, nursery nurses or health care assistants.

The NMC (2008b) Standards introduced the 'sign off' mentor concept so that the final judgement about a student's competence to practise safely is scrutinised by an experienced mentor. The 'sign off' mentor has to undergo additional training and fulfil additional mentorship criteria. The NMC also stipulates that the sign off mentor must:

- Understand the NMC registration requirements.
- Understand the programme requirements and assessment procedures for the students.
- Have been supervised in performing a 'sign off' process of a student on three occasions.
- Have an understanding of their accountability to the NMC when making a decision about student competence and passing practice.

Theoretical foundations and principles

The fifth NMC (2008b) domain for mentors is related to creating a learning environment that is conducive to learning for all learners in the clinical or work setting. A learning environment can be defined as an interactive network of forces within the clinical setting that influence the student's clinical learning outcomes (Stuart, 2007). Creating a good learning environment is the real substance of whether or not learning outcomes are achieved. One way to examine the clinical area could be to perform a SWOT analysis to assess your practice area to see how it might present as an environment for learning. Consider some of the factors that affect the learning environment in Table 2.2 to assist in this exercise.

Protected learning time

Protected learning time (PLT) is used to allow primary healthcare teams time out to learn, protected from service delivery. Different occupational groups have different perceptions and experiences of PLT. Within the nursing field it is viewed as valuable, although in busy environments it can be the first thing to be left out (Cunningham *et al.*, 2006). Protected time is also advocated when mentoring any learner or student nurse in order to fulfil the role effectively (Gopee, 2011). The pace of work and workload in the clinical setting are associated pressures that make it difficult to find time to facilitate learning. However, as team leaders, school nurses will need to facilitate this to ensure that they have full knowledge of the skills and abilities of their team members so that they can effectively address the needs of children, young people and their families.

Tips on how to maximise learning time:

- Think of every experience as a learning one – 'talk as you go', externalise all your thoughts, sharing tacit knowledge.
- Capture all learning opportunities, however minor.
- Try to promote professional conversations with the learner.
- Develop 'case studies' that maybe used to promote understanding.
- Try to have a short 'review' and evaluation session at the end of each day.

Planning teaching/presentations

School nurses may need to teach or present to:

- Young children
- Adolescents
- Parents
- Staff nurses
- Nursery nurses
- Health care assistants
- Other school nurses

Table 2.2 Factors that can affect the learning environment.

Strengths	Weaknesses
■ Effective team leadership	■ Ineffective leadership
■ Updated team members, CPD, extended role	■ Inexperienced or 'out of date' team members
■ An effective working team/flexibility	■ Dysfunctional team
■ Multidisciplinary working	■ Lack of collaboration
■ Well-staffed area with good mentor/learner ratio	■ Staff shortages
■ Well-organised strategies for care delivery, e.g. a philosophy of care	■ Insufficient number of mentors for learners
■ Good communication/record keeping	■ Disorganised care
■ A welcoming atmosphere	■ Poor communication
■ Learner orientation and induction programme	■ Uncomfortable atmosphere and low staff morale
■ Protected time for learners in order to give teaching/feedback	■ No clear orientation programme
■ Study area/quiet room	■ Learners viewed as a hindrance
■ Supernumerary status of learners	■ Learners used as 'workforce'
■ Available learning resources, e.g. care plans, books, journals, policies	■ Limited access to resources
■ Mentorship course	■ No contact with education provider
■ Good links with education provider	■ Learner attitude
■ Learner attitude	
Opportunities	**Threats**
■ Mentorship course	■ Time constraints
■ Personal and professional development	■ Workload
■ Develop teaching skills	■ Change! 'Nothing as constant as change'
■ Leadership	■ Learning not seen as a priority
■ Time to consider good practice and implement things into your area, e.g. Orientation/induction programme for learners	■ Lack of support for learners and learning
■ Multi-professional ways of working	■ Lack of support to do the course
■ Opportunity to scrutinise the care you deliver and your service users	■ Organisation pressures, e.g. reviews, practice theory gaps!
■ Enhance the learning environment	■ Colleagues!
■ Research	■ Learner attitude
■ Audit	

- Teachers
- Other school staff such as learning support assistants
- Conference delegates
- Pre-qualifying nurses
- Student SCPHNs

Within the school nurse setting, a large part of the school nurse's role is related to teaching and learning, either within a group situation or on an individual one-to-one basis (Brown *et al.*, 2011). In both situations it is important that comprehensive planning is done and clarity is sought in every instance to ensure that the target group for each session is made clear. It is not acceptable to take for granted that if you have prepared a session for one group that you could automatically deliver it to a different audience (Walsh, 2010). It is vital that each session is tailor-made and a lesson plan is devised for the intended audience. The types of things that will need to be taken into consideration are the level and age of learner; the content, aims and objectives of the session; and the resources that are available to you (Gopee, 2011). Other constraints, such as the room size, layout, time available and number of learners, are all things you may need to think about when thinking of the learning event that you want to deliver.

When setting aims and objectives for your session try not to fall into the trap of delivering everything that you know about a subject. One of the biggest pitfalls is that of information overload (Walsh, 2010). Start to consider what exactly it is that you intend for your learners to go away with. An aim can be defined as a broad general goal from which you derive more specific objectives. In other words, your aim is your target and your objectives are the steps that you need to take to reach that target.

Objectives are sometimes described using an acronym such as SMART:

- **Specific** – what is expected to be achieved in terms of knowledge and skills.
- **Measurable** – observable and assessable.
- **Achievable** – within the learner's range of abilities.
- **Relevant** – appropriate to the knowledge and skill level expected of the learner.
- **Timed** – clear time-scales set for achievement.

The main objective in professional practice is to impart knowledge and understanding that can then be applied within a work setting (Gopee, 2011). A good lesson plan must therefore incorporate the cognitive, psychomotor and affective aspects of any topic. Bloom's (1956) taxonomy or classifications are useful as a guide to be drawn upon; the three domains are:

- **Cognitive** – knowledge, understanding and comprehension.
- **Psychomotor** – the ' hands on' practical skills.
- **Affective** – the underpinning value judgements and attitudes.

See Activity 2.3 for an activity on planning a teaching session.

Activity 2.3 Planning a teaching session

Think about a teaching session you would like to do.

- What is the aim of your session?
- Consider using Bloom's taxonomy to write your objectives.
- Words to consider when writing objectives:
  - **Cognitive domain** – *name, label, list, select, explain, demonstrate, show, justify, analyse, describe, define, interpret, restate, propose*
  - **Psychomotor domain** – *perform, repeat, arrange, identify, show, calculate, prepare, produce, chart, practise, measure, set up, adapt*
  - **Affective domain** – *evaluate, justify, compare, contrast, challenge, defend, critique*

Remember to consider the level of learner when setting objectives.
(Walsh, 2010)

Other learning opportunities

As well as group teaching, school nurses will also do one-to-one work with children and young people where they will be required to teach. For example, in a drop-in situation, they may be required to teach young people how to safely put on a condom. Bloom's taxonomy can still be applied here because young people need to know the skill of putting the condom on (psychomotor), but they also need the knowledge that school nurses can provide around sexual health and being safe (cognition). The school nurse can also assess the attitude (affective domain) of the young person and make a judgement on their level of maturity (important when considering Fraser competency – see Chapter 6). This may be the only opportunity that the school nurse has to impart knowledge to the young person, as they may only visit once, so it is important to ensure that key messages are received and understood.

Tips on teaching a skill:

- Demonstrate the skill slowly, giving instructions as you do so.
- Demonstrate again without speaking.

- Demonstrate again and ask the young person to tell you what to do.
- Get the young person to do the task and tell you what they are doing.
- Ask them to repeat this again if necessary.

The key messages will be around the practicalities of staying safe, but questions also need to be asked about healthy relationships. This can be an opportunity to open these discussions and give the young person confidence to come back if necessary to talk to the school nurse. This is about establishing trust.

What other key skills will I need?

Understanding child development

This is a huge area, but school nurses should develop their understanding of child development in order for them to make appropriate assessments of children and young people. A fundamental knowledge is essential to understanding behaviours and responding to need. Normally, much of this is taught on the SCPHN course, both in university and in practice, and school nurses should keep updated with any new research. They key areas to be aware of are:

- Developmental milestones (typical and atypical development)
- Attachment theory and how this impacts on the development of relationships and empathy
- The impact of abuse on development
- Transitions and how they will impact on development – for example entering school or changing schools or moving to adult health and social care services
- Resilience theory – what makes some young people more able to cope than others
- The development of the brain and neuroscience across the lifespan
- Understanding adolescence and, in particular, the development of the brain during adolescence

Some useful resources for further reading on these topics are Boushel *et al.* (2000), Gerhardt (2004), Herbert (2003) and Layard and Dunn (2009).

This web page gives good information on the development of the teenage brain: http://www.pbs.org/wgbh/pages/frontline/shows/teenbrain/interviews/giedd.html (accessed 9 March 2012).

Planning care for children with identified needs: developing pathways

The HCP recommends a review of children and young people's health at key points in their lives (see Chapter 7). This is seen as the universal programme and targeted approaches will then focus on children and young people with particular needs. School nurses may be required to be the lead professional in coordinating care as per the Team Around the Child recommendations (TAC, 2012). If they are not the named lead professional, it is important that any care planning is done with school health involvement to ensure that there is a coordinated pathway of care for the child or young person both in school and elsewhere. Some examples of situations where the school nurse may be involved are:

- Asthma
- Epilepsy
- Anaphylaxis
- Diabetes
- Eczema
- Sickle cell disease and thalassaemia

As well as these conditions, school nurses may consider other pathways for young people in their care, for example:

- Young people with alcohol problems
- Young people who are self-harming
- Young people not in school
- Looked after children

A number of terms have been applied to care pathways, but fundamentally they describe the anticipated care for a specific condition, diagnosis or issue over a period of time, and they form part of quality frameworks. The key points are:

- Care pathways are locally developed.
- They should be prepared using the best available evidence.
- They involve agreement through a multidisciplinary team.
- Pathways should be created with user involvement.
- The outcomes are measured through an audit process and reviewed regularly. An expected result should be measured against the actual result (variance analysis).
- Benchmarks can be set in pathways. This is basically setting a standard of excellence which is achievable (SMART indicators can be applied here).
- Care pathways help to demonstrate the effectiveness of services.

See Box 2.1 for an example of good practice in developing pathways of care.

The transfer of information from the early years settings and health visitors to schools and school health teams is crucial for the successful management of

Box 2.1 An exemplar: integrated working; developing protocols and care pathways

A 0–19 integrated nursing team (comprising school nurses, health visitors, community staff nurses, nursery nurses and healthcare support workers) in the North of England identified a need to 'streamline and rationalise' the planning of care for children and young people across the different localities in the area. There were three particular areas of focus: protocols for care plans for children with additional or complex needs, children missing education and delivery of drop-ins in the High Schools in the area. Student SCPHN (school nurses) were involved in these projects in setting up audit tools, disseminating information to school nurse forums and collating questionnaires in the drop-in research.

1. Care plan protocols

It was recognised that there was some variation in the approach to developing care plans for children with additional or complex needs across the localities. The care plan protocol was developed in partnership with key stakeholders to ensure that 0–19 team members were clear on the processes for instigating, developing and reviewing health care plans that serve to assist schools in safely supporting children and young people who have long term medical needs.

The care plan protocol includes:

- A rationale for developing the protocol and the key principles that guide it.
- The roles and responsibilities of those involved in care delivery.
- The procedure for developing and reviewing the care plan.
- Guidance on completion and storage of records: all now held electronically and reviewed annually (or sooner if changes occur).
- The identification of any training needs of staff.
- Care plan templates for recording the child/young person's details and the care given.
- Letter templates to parents to invite comment/information on any changes at the annual review and a reminder letter for non-responses.

The Trust has a Quality Improvement Framework which is set and reviewed annually. For 2011–2012 the care plan protocol will be reviewed under the patient-centred care domain. Adherence to the protocol will be audited with a particular focus on how well children/young people and their families are involved in their own care. One of the SCPHN student school nurses (with help from the other students and a Practice Teacher) will lead on developing an audit tool to perform this task. They will then analyse the results and develop an action plan producing a final report and implementing any recommendations from this.

2. Children missing education

Clinical leaders from within the school nursing team worked with a multidisciplinary group of key stakeholders from health and education to agree a pathway for identification, communication and support for any children who are missing from education (CME), in line with local safeguarding policies and procedures.

The aim was to ensure that children who are not receiving, or at risk of not receiving, a suitable education are identified quickly, and arrangements put in place to assess their health needs and provide intervention where necessary.

It was also aimed at promoting children's health and wellbeing through effective collaboration, communication and information sharing between agencies so that coordinated and comprehensive services for CME can be planned and implemented.

The protocol included:

- The rationale for the protocol and the identification of the need for a Children Missing from Education (CME) team.
- Clear descriptions of the roles and responsibilities of all those involved: CME team, school nurse, A&E liaison nurse, administration staff, school and safeguarding team.
- An integrated pathway describing the communication strategy for reporting and tracking CME.
- Clear routes to guide reporting of missing children to the local police.
- The use of 'hyperlinks' to secure NHS links to communicate referrals.
- Template forms for recording and sharing information.
- An algorithm to clarify the process.

3. High school drop-in: 'setting a benchmark'

This project aimed to review the drop-in services that were available in secondary schools in the area, gain the views of children and young people and assess the uptake of these services. A scoping exercise was conducted to determine the number of schools offering drop-ins across the area. A questionnaire was compiled and sent to pupils in five of the secondary schools where drop-ins were offered. The views of school nurses were also recorded. Although those young people who accessed the service found it valuable, the results demonstrated a poor uptake of the services, mainly due to poor marketing strategies (few pupils knew about the service). The scoping exercise also showed that not all schools had access to a drop-in.

The recommendations from the research were to:

- Actively market the benefits of drop-in services and develop drop-in services in schools where there were none.
- Improve awareness of the service in schools where there was a service, through advertising, posters and attending assemblies.
- Improve communication via more collaborative working with PHSE coordinators, pastoral support, Heads of Year and the safeguarding named teacher.
- Vary the methods of communication with pupils, e.g. school web pages, email, texting, message box.
- Consider the place and time for the drop-in to actively improve ease of access.
- Every team to have at least one member who has undertaken accredited PSHE course training to act as resource and provide leadership.

The benchmark group responsible in the area for measuring quality and standards set a benchmark for practice which aimed to measure the standard of service delivered through the school nurse-led drop-in service within educational settings, and the level to which school nurses are prepared for this role. The findings from the benchmarking exercise were very similar to those gained from the student survey and reaffirmed the recommendations above with the addition of two further recommendations:

- Develop a standard operating procedure to guide and standardise the delivery of drop-ins with a formal audit undertaken to monitor and improve practice.
- Develop a single documentation sheet for all school nurses to use when undertaking a drop-in session.

An action plan was developed to support implementation of the recommendations all of which are now implemented or in progress. A further drop-in questionnaire is planned to evaluate progress.

The integrated team consists of Lynn Pinder, school nurse and practice teacher, and members of the school nursing team and school nursing students who contributed to the development and implementation of this work.

children with identified needs and is a recommendation in the HCP (DH/DCSF, 2009). Some areas have integrated 0–19 teams to ensure this smooth transition of information (see Box 2.1).

There may be situations where a child or young person has a complex health need where they may be too ill to attend school or they may attend a special school where there is a nurse attached to the school permanently. These children and young people will have specific care plans or pathways and the role of the nurse may be a clinical one, which will be clearly defined; they may not be SCPHN trained. Working in partnership with these teams, however, is still important to address the other needs of these children and young people (such as their emotional and social needs). Giving support to these nurses and providing multi-agency care pathways will be important here.

Nurses in special schools can feel isolated from other community teams and have expressed concerns that they are often forgotten when study days are planned. They find it difficult to take time out to attend important updates and qualified SCPHNs, as leaders of the school health teams, should be keeping lines of communication open and be inclusive.

Schools and their employers should have policies on managing pupils' medicines and on supporting pupils with medical needs, and school nurses should be involved in these policies. The *Managing Medicines in Schools and Early Years Settings* document(DH/DfES, 2005) provides good resources with excellent templates for recording individualised care.

The coordination of care should involve all relevant people involved in the child's or young person's life, with a clear focus on the wishes of the child and their parents or carers. The school nurse role may also be around training staff and others about specific conditions and they should work closely with parents to ensure that there is full understanding of a child's or young person's individual needs.

Consideration should also be given to the transition from school into the workplace for young people with complex needs. In some areas, transition nurses have been employed to address the gaps in these services and coordinate this care, but in others it may be a role for school nurses in partnership with community children's nurses, particularly as the Healthy Child Programme continues until the 20th birthday (DH/DCSF, 2009).

Clinical nursing skills

Part of the uniqueness of school nursing is that while a public health role, some clinical skills are still maintained. Two key examples of this are in the assessment of children with particular health needs (as above) and in the immunisation programmes that they deliver. Although in some areas immunisation teams have been formed, school nurses are still involved in this important public health work. As team leaders, school nurses will need to ensure that the team is appropriately trained to immunise safely. They will be responsible for ensuring that the team is competent and the Health Protection Agency (HPA, 2005) has produced guidelines for national minimum standards for immunisation training.

In summary, these guidelines state that:

1. Anyone who immunises or advises on immunisations should be on a relevant professional register, such as the NMC, GMC or equivalent.
2. Anyone who immunises or advises on immunisations should attend regular updates and receive specific training. Those new to immunising should be supervised by an experienced immuniser and attend a formal taught course at the earliest opportunity.
3. The content of training should include:
   (a) The aims of immunisation: national policy and schedules.
   (b) The immune system and how vaccines work.
   (c) Vaccine preventable diseases.
   (d) The different types of vaccine and their composition.
   (e) Current issues and controversies regarding immunisation.
   (f) Communicating with patients, parents and young people.
   (g) Legal aspects of vaccination (including consent).
   (h) Storage and handling of vaccines.
   (i) Correct administration of vaccines.
   (j) Anaphylaxis and other adverse events.
   (k) Documentation, record keeping and reporting.
   (l) Strategies for improving immunisation rates.
4. The minimum duration of basic training should be two days. Annual updates must be provided for and attended by those who have attended basic training.
5. Anyone who is immunising should have access to the 'Green Book' (DH, 2006a) and all updates of national vaccinations policy including any CNO/CMO/CPO letters.
6. Those responsible for quality and clinical governance should ensure that staff training is included in regular audit of the immunisation service.

School nurses involved in immunisation sessions will need to be aware of critical incident forms should there be a problem (such as an immunisation error or an adverse reaction to the immunisation) at a session. Critical incidents will have to be reported locally and there will be procedures in place for this. The potential critical incidents include:

- No informed consent
- The wrong form with the wrong child
- The wrong vaccine
- Accidental overdose of the vaccine
- Out-of-date vaccine
- Incorrect interval between vaccines
- A needle stick injury
- An anaphylactic reaction to the vaccine
- Any other adverse reaction to the vaccine

To minimise the potential for errors, here is a checklist:

1. Check the local policy for health and safety guidance.
2. Make sure you have the patient group direction (PGD) and the Green Book at the session to refer to if necessary.
3. Ensure that there is epinephrine available, in date, for any anaphylactic reactions.
4. Have an individual 'station' for each nurse.
5. Each nurse should draw up their own vaccines for administration and check each one for date etc. with a colleague.
6. Sharps boxes need to be correctly assembled, one for each nurse. Do not share sharps boxes.
7. The young person should be sitting down in front of you (not standing).
8. Ensure there is not an 'audience' of other children – those waiting should be out of sight.
9. Carefully check the form. Ask the young person's name and check that the form is signed.
10. Ask the appropriate questions for the vaccine being given (e.g. are they unwell, pregnant etc.). Have a checklist with you to remind you of the contra-indications as well as the Green Book.

Any adverse reactions to the vaccine should be reported via The 'Yellow Card Scheme'. This is run by the Medicines and Healthcare Products Regulatory Agency (MHRA), a government agency responsible for ensuring that medicines and medical devices work and are acceptably safe. The system is jointly run with the Commission on Human Medicines (CHM), and is used to collect information from both health professionals and the general public on suspected side effects or adverse reactions to a medicine. Yellow cards can be sent in by anyone from the UK on both licensed and unlicensed medicines including:

- Prescription medicines
- Vaccines
- Over-the-counter (OTC) medicines
- Herbal remedies
- Swine flu antiviral medicines (Tamiflu or Relenza)
- Swine flu vaccines (Pandemrix, made by GSK or Celvapan, made by Baxter)

Record keeping

Accurate record keeping and documentation are important in professional practice. Once something is written down, it is a permanent account of what has happened and also what has been said. Remember, if it is not written down there is a sense that somehow 'it didn't happen'. Without a written record of events there is no evidence to support a decision made or an audit trail from which to follow a sequence of events. It is therefore crucial that accurate and consistent records are kept at all times. The *Guidelines for Records and Record Keeping* (NMC, 2002, p. 2), state clearly that:

> the quality of your record keeping is also a reflection of the standard of your professional practice. Good record keeping is a mark of the skilled and safe practitioner, whilst careless or incomplete record keeping often highlights wider problems with the individual's practice

The obligation from the above statement is clear that professionally, nurses are accountable for keeping accurate and consistent records. When it comes to making good quality records they should be:

- Clear and accurate
- Factual, consistent, and relevant
- Comprehensive and useful
- Contemporaneous (made at the time)

The NHS is now moving towards paper-free record keeping and installing IT systems to facilitate this. The RiO system is the central spine of this technology across the country, with the intention that all areas of the NHS will use this electronic database to store records safely. Uptake of this has been slow and sporadic, but ultimately, in this modern age, the use of technology looks set to continue.

The other element of accurate record keeping relates closely to investigations and serious untoward incidents (SUI) (DH, 2006b). The principal definition of an SUI is:

... something out of the ordinary or unexpected, with the potential to cause serious harm, that is likely to attract public and media interest that occurs on NHS premises or in the provision of an NHS or a commissioned service. SUIs are not exclusively clinical issues, for example, an electrical failure may have consequences that make it an SUI. (NHS, 2009).

School nurses have been involved in critical incidents in the past relating to information that they have given to young people in PSHE lessons or about giving sexual health or contraceptive advice to young people under 16. In this respect, it is important that there is confidence in the protocols and guidance that are in place to guide practitioners, that practitioners have adhered to them and that local communication teams are involved if the incident is likely to be in the media.

Organisational skills

The key to being organised is to:

- Prepare well in advance and identify the required resources for the planned task, project or meeting.
- Be realistic about how long a task or project will take – for school nurses, this will include estimating travel times.
- Develop a timetable of events and tasks with deadlines and reminders embedded. Use technology to your advantage as we move towards a 'paper-free world'. If you are not a naturally organised person, technology can be really helpful, as electronic devices now have organisers which will prompt you when something is due and you can set reminders for days or weeks before, as required. Take the time to learn how to do this and set time aside each week to update your task list, this will save time in the long run. Make sure information is backed up to another device in case of a technical failure.
- Arrange tasks in a logical order of priority, with urgent matters dealt with first. Be wary that 'unimportant tasks' may be forgotten, so take care to revisit these tasks when there is time.
- Allow space and time for unplanned events to occur each day. If there is not a problem, you can then tackle the less important tasks in your 'to do' list.

Conclusion

In summary, this chapter has considered some of the key skills that school nurses need to be effective in their role. It is clear that the remit of the school nurse has the potential to be extensive and utilising the knowledge and skills across teams is vital as resources are limited. As leaders, school nurses should identify the most appropriate people for particular roles. They also need to work in close partnership with other agencies to best serve the needs of young people and their families. The unique skills of the qualified school nurse centre around their leadership qualities, their ability to assess need and their skill in communicating the needs of children and young people to a broader audience. They form a vital link between health, education and social services and are a first point of contact for many young people.

References

Agenda for Change (2012) *How Agenda for Change Works*. Available at http://www.nh-semployers.org/PayAndContracts/AgendaForChange/Pages/Afc-AtAGlanceRP.aspx (accessed 17 January 2012).

Ancona,D., Malone, T. W., Orlikowski,W. J. and Senge, P. (2007) In praise of the incomplete leader. *Harvard Business Review*, **85**(2), 92–100.

Aveyard, H. (2010) *Doing a Literature Review in Health and Social Care*, 2nd edn. McGraw-Hill, Berkshire.

Bloom,B. (1956) *Taxonomy of Educational Objectives: The Classification of Educational Goals, Handbook One: Cognitive Domain*. Longman, London.

Brown, J., Busfield, R., O'Shea, A. and Sibthorpe, J. (2011) School ethos and personal, social, health education. *Pastoral Care in Education*, **29**(2), 117–31.

Boud, D., Keough, R. and Walker, D. (1985) *Reflection: Turning Experience Into Learning*. Kogan, London.

Boushel, M., Fawcett, M. and Selwyn, J. (2000) *Focus on Early Childhood: Principles and Realities*. Blackwell Science, Oxford.

Cronin, P., Ryan, F. and Coughlan, M. (2008) Undertaking a literature review- a step by step approach. *British Journal of Nursing*, **17**(1), 38–43.

Cunningham, D., Fitzpatrick, B. and Kelly, D. (2006) Practice managers' perceptions and experiences of protected learning time: a focus group study. *Quality in Primary Care*, **14**, 169–75.

Department of Health/Department for Education and Skills (2005) *Managing Medicines in Schools and Early Years Settings*. Available at http://www.education.gov.uk/schools/pupilsupport/pastoralcare/b0013771/managing-medicines-in-schools (accessed 9 March 2012).

Department of Health (2006a) *Immunisation Against Infectious Disease (The Green Book)*. Available at http://www.dh.gov.uk/en/Publichealth/Immunisation/Greenbook/ (accessed 9 March 2012).

Department of Health (2006b) *Safeguarding Children and Young People: Roles and Competences for Health Care Staff, Intercollegiate Document*. DH, London.

Department of Health/Department for Children, Schools and Families (2009) *The Healthy Child Programme from 5 to 19*. DH/DCSF, London.

Department of Health (2012) *Getting it Right for Children, Young People and Their Families. Maximising the Contribution of the School Nursing Team. Vision and Call to Action*. DH, London.

Fink, A. (2005) *Conducting Research Literature Reviews 'From the Internet to Paper'*. Sage, London.

Fisher, R. and Ury, W. (2003) *Getting to Yes – Negotiating an Agreement Without Giving In*. Random House Business Books, London.

Gates, S. (2011) *The Negotiation Book: Your Definitive Guide to Successful Negotiation*. John Wiley & Sons, Chichester.

Gerhardt, S. (2004) *Why Love Matters: How Affection Shapes a Baby's Brain*. Brunner-Routledge, Hove.

Ghaye, T. (2011) *Teaching and Learning Through Reflective Practice: A Practical Guide for Positive Action Learning*, 2nd edn. Routledge, Oxfordshire.

Gopee, N. (2011) *Mentoring and Supervision in Healthcare*, 2nd edn. Sage, London.

Gray, D. (2004) *Doing Research in the Real World*. Sage, London.

Health Protection Agency (2005) *National Minimum Standards for Immunisation Training*. HPA, London.

Herbert, M. (2003) *Typical and Atypical Development: From Conception to Adolescence*. Blackwell, Oxford.

Ironside, V. (2004) *The Huge Bag of Worries*. Hodder Children's Books, London.

Johns, C. (1992) The Burford nursing development unit holistic model of nursing practice. *Journal of Advanced Nursing*, **16**, 1090–8.

Layard, R. and Dunn, J. (2009) *A Good Childhood*. The Children's Society/Penguin Books, London.

Martin, V., Charelsworth, J. and Henderson, E. (2010) *Managing in Health and Social Care*, 2nd edn. Routledge, London.

KSF Guidelines (2010) *Appraisals and KSF Made Simple, a Practical Guide*. Available at http://www.nhsemployers.org/Aboutus/Publications/Pages/AppraisalsAndKSFMadeSimple-ApracticalGuide.aspx (accessed 17 January 2012).

NHS Executive (1993) *A Vision for the Future; Report of the Chief Nursing Officer*. London, NHSE.

NHS London (2009) *Serious Untoward Incident Reporting Policy Including the Procedure to Be Followed for Safguarding Children*. NHS, London.

Nursing and Midwifery Council (2002) *Guidelines for Records and Record Keeping*. NMC, London.

Nursing and Midwifery Council (2008a) *The Code: Standards of Conduct, Performance and Ethics for Nurses and Midwives*. NMC, London.

Nursing and Midwifery Council (2008b) *Standards to Support Learning and Assessment in Practice*. NMC, London.

Nursing and Midwifery Council (2011a) *The Prep Handbook*. NMC, London.

Nursing and Midwifery Council (2011b) *Supporting and Assessing Learning in Practice – the Practice Teacher Role*. NMC, London.

Ogier, M. (1989) *Working and Learning*. Scutari Press, London.

Parahoo, K. (2006) *Nursing Research: Principles, Process and Issues*, 2nd edn. Palgrave Macmillan, Hampshire.

Peberdy, D. and Hammersley, J. (2009) *Brilliant Meetings: What to Know, Say and Do to Have Fewer, Better Meetings*. Pearson Education, Edinburgh.

Quinn, F. M. (2008) *The Principles and Practice of Nurse Education*, 4th edn. Stanley Thornes, Cheltenham.

Ramsbottom, O., Woodhouse, T. and Miall, H. (2011) *Contemporary Conflict Resolution*, 3rd edn. Polity Press, Malden.

Rogers, C. (1956) *Client-Centred Therapy*. Constable and Company, London.

Stewart, R. (1989*) Leading in the NHS: A Practical Guide*. Macmillan, London.

Stuart, C.C. (2007) *Assessment, Supervision and Support in Clinical Practice*. Churchill Livingstone, London.

Taylor, C. and White, S. (2000) *Practising Reflexivity in Health and Welfare: Making Knowledge*. Open University Press, Buckingham.

Team Around the Child [TAC] (2012) *The Team Around the Child*. Available at http://www. education.gov.uk/childrenandyoungpeople/strategy/integratedworking/a0068944/ team-around-the-child-tac (accessed 8 January 2012).

Tyler, S. (2004) *The Manager's Good Study Guide: An Essential Reference with Key Concepts, Tools and Techniques Explained*, 3rd edn. Open University Press, Milton Keynes.

Walsh, D. (2010) *The Nurse Mentor's Handbook – Supporting Students in Clinical Practice*. Open University Press, Maidenhead.

Walshe, K. and Smith, J. (2011) *Healthcare Management*, 2nd edn. McGraw-Hill, London.

Wood, S. (1998) Ethics and communication: developing reflective practice. *Nursing Standard*, **12**(18), 44–7.

Yoder-Wise, P. (2011) *Leading and Managing in Nursing*, 5th edn. Elsevier, New York.

CHAPTER 3

Dealing with difficult situations

Jane Wright and Lynne Smith

Key themes in this chapter:

- Section 1: Difficult issues in the workplace
  - How do I deal with difficult teams or team members?
  - What do I do if I feel that I am being bullied?
  - How do I prioritise my work?
  - Coping with workload stress.
- Section 2: Working with children, young people and their families
  - How do I deal with a child that is bullied?
  - How do I deal with young victims who do not know that they are being abused?
  - How do I deal with children and young people who self-harm?
  - What about children and young people who are abusing substances?
  - How do I reach disadvantaged or marginalised groups?
  - How do I respond to looked after children's needs?

Introduction

This chapter explores issues around dealing with difficult situations. It is divided into two sections. The first section looks at issues related to workload, staff/team issues and personal difficulties. The second section looks at the types of problem that school nurses encounter with children, young people and families. There are case studies throughout this chapter to illustrate issues that have been identified through talking to a number of practitioners about the difficulties they have faced as a Specialist Community Public Health Nurse (SCPHN). All names have been changed to protect anonymity.

Section 1: Difficult issues in the workplace

How do I deal with difficult teams or team members?

Newly-qualified school nurses may be faced with the new experience of leading difficult teams. This may be a particular problem if you are trying to make a change to practice. Students completing the SCPHN course are enthused to make changes because they study current research, practice and theory as well as leadership and management skills. They have also had opportunities to look at practice from different perspectives and in different areas and this means that they are motivated to consider best practice and raise the profile of school nursing.

Forming teams

Although you may be joining an already established team, it is important to form your own team and establish group cohesion quickly (see Case study 3.1).

Case study 3.1

Following my qualification as a school nurse I got a job leading a team of three, including a community staff nurse and two nursery nurses. From the outset there was an atmosphere of clear resentment of my new role as a SCPHN. I had been a community staff nurse (CSN) in the same area before doing the degree and I got the feeling that there was a problem with them thinking that I had got 'above myself'. I decided that the best way to deal with this was to establish from the outset that I was no longer a CSN and that I would be leading the team, but that I would need their support to do this.

I called a team meeting early on, followed by individual private meetings with all of them. At the team meeting I asked them outright to air their views, expectations, resentments and issues and that this was their chance to do this. They were surprised by this development and were brave enough to say what they felt. The resentment seemed to come from a lack of support for them in the past and that the CSN had not got the sponsorship to do the course I had just finished. I allowed them to be honest about all of this and then told them that this was a new way of working where their views would be listened to on a regular basis and that I would support their continuing professional development. We then made a plan together about what the vision for the team was, how we were going to achieve it and what each

> of our roles were. We made a 'contract' which we all agreed to. A weekly team meeting was agreed for early on a Monday morning.
>
> I then met each of the team individually to identify any individual problems and establish what they wanted in terms of CPD.
>
> All this worked well. The team had felt able to say what they thought openly and we were able to move forward as a team.

Tuckman (Business Balls, 2011) outlined key stages in the formation of teams which are relevant here:

- **Forming**: Although there may be an established team, this is still a new era with a new leader and this forming stage is important; a new leader may be seen to challenge the norms and dynamics of a group and cause anxiety. This may be an initially comfortable stage where people are getting to know each other and are keen to discover what the future of the team may be. They may not fully reveal themselves until the goals are established. This can be a very short period of time or it can take some time.
- **Storming**: Tuckman argues that every group will go through this storming stage in their development. This is where different ideas from members of the group may compete for consideration. Conflict may occur in this stage, as members of the team may have fixed ideas about the direction in which the school nursing service should be going, for example. Alternatively, the team may not want change because it is content with how things are and cannot see a clear reason for any change. Acceptance or non-acceptance of the leader will occur at this stage of the team's development, and therefore it is a crucial time for a new team leader. If this stage can be resolved quickly, then the team can move forward; if not, the group may never move out of this potentially chaotic period of development. There seems to be some agreement among theorists that this stage is necessary for the growth of the team, and although it can be an unpleasant time, it is the opportunity for members of the team to express their views and feelings. The leader here must be tolerant of the views of the members, show patience and be non-judgemental. Active listening is a key skill here (see Chapter 2). It may also be a time, however, that the leader needs to imprint their control over the group. Listening to ideas is fine, but the leader should also consider the greater issues within school nursing practice, such as the political agenda. This may mean that changes have to be made regardless of how people feel them.

- **Norming**: This stage may never be reached, but it is hoped that the team will develop and agree a common goal. This may involve a compromise from all members of the team and a leader should be prepared to do this while maintaining the integrity of the main changes that they want to make. Negotiation on less important parts of the plan may be necessary at this stage, but of course they could be revisited later.

- **Performing**: If a team can reach this stage, then it can become efficient, cohesive and autonomous. The aim is to have a highly-motivated, competent and confident group where members have clearly defined roles which complement each other to achieve the common purpose. Dissent may be expected within teams, and they should not operate without members questioning what is expected of them – this should be actively encouraged. Challenging practice and using best evidence is embedded within nursing and nurses are, of course, accountable for their actions at all times (NMC, 2008). Members of the team should know the processes that are in place to protect both them and the members of the public, and the leader must be approachable as well as knowledgeable. The process of forming teams is not fixed once this stage is reached – it is more cyclical, reverting back to the storming stage from time to time.

- **Adjourning**: This fifth stage was added later by Jenson (Business Balls, 2011). It is considered the stage where the task is finished and the group is disbanded. Where school nurse teams work within a larger team, for example in immunisation teams, this may be a relevant stage to be aware of as a phase of readjustment and reorientation.

Leadership

There is a difference between management and leadership and both have a role to play in understanding teams. One view is that while management is about processes and functions, leadership is about behaviours and relationships. An example of the difference may be seen if we consider a military battle. The 'manager' will plan the battle on paper, measuring and assessing the capabilities of the soldiers or troops, and examining their potential and particular strengths. The manager would then make decisions based on this information (a good manager uses the best people for the job) and then communicate the intentions to the relevant people. This uses the organisation's systems and processes to assess the best course of action in a given situation.

The one who actually leads people into battle may use some of these skills, but must possess something less tangible in order for the soldiers to follow them into a dangerous situation. These qualities include trust, inspiration, respect, honesty and decision-making skills.

Leadership traits

- **Integrity and honesty**: this implies that you can trust the decisions that are made and that this person will be true to what they say; they will be reliable and truthful.
- **Humility**: this implies that the leader is unassuming and modest and has the whole team's interest at heart and not just their own status or future. Team members need to feel safe in the hands of their leader in order to function effectively.
- **Courage**: having the courage to make difficult decisions is crucial. A team will need to feel confident that a leader will make these decisions in the best interest of the team goals.
- **Commitment**: a committed leader is one who leads by example and is always accessible and visible.
- **Sincerity**: team members need to believe what the leader says.
- **Passion**: a really important trait in school nursing. Team leaders need to be passionate about the service and the team needs to be confident that the leader is not just 'passing through' the service but will drive forward the ideas of the team.
- **Confidence**: self-confidence is important when making decisions and also when running meetings. A confident and assertive leader will inspire the confidence in others.
- **Assertiveness**: alongside confidence is assertiveness. As leaders, school nurses need to ensure that they act as advocates for school nursing practice in different settings. This may be with managers, with commissioners, at conferences or at other stakeholder meetings.
- **Optimism**: a negative leader will not inspire any confidence in the team and a disillusioned team will not function well. Maintaining the morale of a team is really important, particularly when there are times of political unrest, economic uncertainty or limited resources.
- **Wisdom**: leaders should be knowledgeable and contemporary in their approach. This means they need to keep up to date with the ever-changing political agenda as well as understanding how to raise the profile of school nursing in a local and broader context.
- **Determination**: a determined leader will ensure that the team is listened to and that team goals are reached. Take care though that the goals are not the individual leader's own personal ones.

- **Compassion**: leaders need to understand the team members and show concern and kindness when necessary. Understanding that people have personal lives which will occasionally impact on their work is very important. This obviously needs to be balanced against considering the service as a whole and the young people who depend upon it.
- **Charisma**: this is difficult to quantify but relates to charm and personality. People with charisma can sometimes become leaders without expecting to because of this.

Managing change

Change is perhaps the most difficult thing to deal with in terms of leading a team. A leader may face difficulties with this when a team has been functioning for some time and view the new team leader with some scepticism or suspicion.

Change theories

Kurt Lewin's force field theory (Lewin, 1951):

Lewin's theory considers the process of behaviour change as being related to forces which affect the equilibrium of either individuals or groups. In particular, two forces are involved in change: the restraining force and the driving force. A shift or change will naturally go in the direction of the stronger force; therefore, if the driving force is strong enough, change will occur. He considered the first step to change is to introduce a force which alters the status quo or balance. This maps to Tuckman's view of 'storming' within a new group, where there is an inevitable shift, however small, in the equilibrium of a group. If you alter the 'natural state' by introducing a force (such as heat on ice) then you change the overall shape and identity of the structure and create movement. Once you have movement, you can then reshape the structure to a new form, such as moulding clay into a pot. 'Unfreezing' a situation requires three steps, the first is to increase the driving force that will persuade others that change is needed. This could be a change in the political agenda for example; for school nurses, this will 'unbalance' teams and force them to make change. The second step of unfreezing is to remove the barriers to change or decrease the restraining forces. Essentially, this means making the process easier; being clear about the new objectives, being positive about the change and reassuring staff about their jobs. Building the team during the movement phase involves motivating them and encouraging them to look at different perspectives. Understanding group dynamics, then, is important in managing change.

Resisting forces from individuals:

- Fear of the unknown
- Lack of confidence in own or others' ability
- Previous experience of poor change management
- Has experienced a lot of change already
- A lack of cohesion in the team
- Dislike or distrust of the leader
- A communication difficulty, such as Asperger's or autistic spectrum
- Attention Deficit Hyperactivity Disorder (ADHD) tendencies
- A mental health problem such as depression
- Personality type – the 'big five' personality traits have been described as OCEAN:
  - Open/closed
  - Conscientiousness/non-conscientious
  - Extrovert/introvert
  - Agreeable/non-agreeable
  - Neurotic/stable

(Costa and McCrae, 1992)

The Myers–Briggs Type Indicator (MBTI) is a psychometric assessment of personality and is often used in the workplace to identify how people interact with each other and what potential conflicts may be present (MBTI, 2012). The MBTI can also be helpful to identify what kind of leader you are.

Those most likely to resist change will be those who have a closed, introverted or neurotic personality. A non-agreeable personality may also look suspiciously on change and could also be antagonistic to the team members. This can be linked to Belbin's theory around team member types (Belbin, 1981).

Belbin's team members types:

- **Coordinator (Extrovert).** This is a leader who is able to motivate others towards a common aim – they are confident and mature.
- **Shaper (Extrovert).** The shaper of the group is motivated, enthusiastic, assertive and competitive.
- **Plant (Extrovert).** The plant is the creative member of the group who comes up with good ideas as to how to get something done, not always conventional.
- **Monitor–Evaluator (Introvert).** The monitor–evaluator is the person who thinks things through critically and assesses the situation in a thoughtful way.
- **Implementer (Introvert/Conscientious).** This person is the dependable one who will implement the ideas in a sensible way. They are reliable and apply common sense to the situation.

- **Resource investigator (Conscientious/Agreeable)**. The resource investigator will look at how things can be achieved, they will look at options and are good communicators and negotiators.
- **Team worker (Agreeable)**. The team worker can be the mediator or calming influence; they are usually affable and sociable.
- **Completer/finisher (Conscientious)**. The completer/finisher is orientated towards quality and standards and will ensure that the tasks are completed to a high specification.
- **Specialist (Closed)**. Highly focused on their area; may have a very specific area of interest and is driven by professionalism

The role of the team leader will be to understand the individual members of the team, what their skills are and how to get the best performance from them. Also, how to deal with problems as they arise is key. Clear protocols for managing staff should be available and staff appraisals used to identify strengths and areas for development. Appraisals are discussed in Chapter 2. What is expected of each team member should be clearly identified and all members of the team should feel they are able to approach you with problems. Once they do, you need to act straight away.

What types of problem might I encounter with staff?
- Regular lateness
- Regular sickness
- Depression or other emotional problems
- Mental health problems such as a personality disorder
- Attitude problems (difficult to measure)
- Overt aggression/anger/resentment
- Passive aggression. There might be individuals who will undermine your leadership in subtle ways while appearing to be very supportive.
- Emotional outbursts (e.g. crying in meetings)
- Complaints from schools or parents about communication skills
- Contacting you at inappropriate times, for example at home during the evening or at the weekend
- Becoming dependent on you for support for personal matters rather than work issues
- Breaching confidentiality
- Inappropriate dress
- Hygiene issues
- Alcoholism

- Substance misuse
- Trying to work too fast and making mistakes
- Relationships between members of the team either positive or negative
- A personal problem that is affecting their work (see Case study 3.2)

Case study 3.2

Following taking over as a team leader of three staff members (one administrator, a nursery nurse and a community staff nurse) it became clear that the nursery nurse was experiencing real emotional problems at home and this was impacting on her work. Unfortunately, she lost her temper in a school and shouted at a group of students, who consequently complained, as did their parents.

I arranged to meet with her and discuss the problems informally to establish what the problems were. She was very upset and had been having some problems at home with her partner who, it transpired was leaving her. It is really difficult getting a balance between being sympathetic while maintaining a professional boundary and considering the service's needs.

I allowed her to talk and then to identify for herself how she could cope with the home problems as well as work. She decided she would take two weeks off as sick leave where she would visit her GP and seek some counselling help, and then we made an action plan for her return. I felt it was necessary to meet with her each week to monitor her progress following her return and made it clear that any similar behaviour would not be tolerated in the future. We then recorded our conversation and signed an action plan.

I had to cover her two weeks off and talk to the rest of the team about this without breaching her confidence. On her return, we phased her visits into schools and ensured that, initially, she was with other members of the team. She did very well and no further incidents were reported.

Remember, the NMC recommends that new employees should have:

- A thorough induction into their area of work
- Training and supervision where necessary
- Preceptorship and mentoring (especially for newly-qualified staff)
- Ongoing access to professional development
- Clinical supervision
  (NMC, 2011)

The Human Resources department is there to give advice and support and to take on particular problems if necessary. Good protocols and policies are also important for transparency. Do not become a bully yourself (see next section); ensure that an employee does not feel victimised or intimidated. To do this you need to remain professional at all times and treat everyone in the same way:

- Have good, indisputable policies and procedures in place and if they are not there already, create them.
- Be decisive; make clear decisions and keep to them.
- Don't discuss individuals with other members of the team.
- Don't give out home numbers to colleagues – they should have no need to contact you at home. Management or the HR department will have your home number for an emergency.
- Be wary of becoming friends with team members. It can lead to problems; remember you are the leader. This does not mean that you cannot be 'friendly'.
- Treat everyone fairly, i.e. in the same way.
- Be a role model: turn up early for meetings, always do what you say you are going to do and maintain the confidence of all staff. You cannot expect the team to do these things if you don't.
- Consider the boundaries needed for leadership. Don't display favouritism to individuals however much you like them because you will alienate other members of the team.
- Be sympathetic to personal problems but be wary of becoming too involved other than giving time off or referring them to other help via occupational health. You are not there to be an emotional crutch.
- Give everyone a chance to speak at meetings to air their views (see Chapter 2).
- Show respect to the views of your team but be clear about the promotion of anti-discriminatory behaviour and language.

Giving informal feedback

Talk to the individual privately as soon as possible after identifying the problem/s. It is a mistake to allow an issue to go on for too long, this can reinforce the behaviour and in turn condone it. The problem or behaviour may then become entrenched.

Where possible tell the individual what it is you are going to discuss before a meeting. This will reduce the stress levels of the individual even if the problem is a difficult one.

- Consult with Human Resources on the procedure.

- Be careful about 'collecting' information before seeing the individual, because this will look to them as though you are making a case against them and will cause antagonism.
- Be sensitive to when the most appropriate time to talk is – for example, not on a Friday, which may result in individuals being upset over a weekend. They may be on their own, and talking earlier in the week will allow them time to talk at work if they want to.
- Make space and time in private for the meeting, away from a phone that may ring or where other people may listen.
- Be honest and clear about what the problem is.
- Consider basic communication skills such as body language – making eye contact etc. (see Chapter 2).
- Find something positive to say about the person. However difficult the problem is, there is always something that they have done well, however small.
- Ensure that the individual feels they are contributing to the solutions; they are more likely to comply if they have helped set the agenda.
- Be transparent about what you are going to do and what the protocols are.
- Make clear decisions so that individuals know what is expected of both them and you.
- Finish the meeting with a written action plan which includes achievable goals for both you and the individual and set another date to review it formally.
- Ensure there is a third party present if the issue is very serious (for example a professional issue such as breaching confidentiality or a complaint), because disciplinary procedures may be needed.
- Record keeping – make sure you document everything that is done.

Grievances or disciplinary action

The Arbitration, Conciliation and Advisory service (ACAS) provides a code of practice for raising both grievances and disciplinary procedures (ACAS, 2009). The code suggests that a mediator, either internal or external, should be used in cases where informal meetings have failed to satisfy either party (either the employee or the employer). Disciplinary procedures are used for misconduct or poor performance and grievances are concerns, problems or complaints from an employee. Fairness and transparency are key to the procedures that are in place locally to deal with both grievances and disciplinary action. The code of practice suggests that employees are involved in the creation of these rules and procedures and that they are easily accessible to the staff (ACAS, 2009). This gives ownership to the workforce and can also be applied to other protocols and procedures used in the workplace.

Employers have to be seen to act fairly in these situations, and the key elements to this are:

- Act promptly, avoid unreasonable delays.
- Act consistently.
- Establish the facts of the case fairly; this may involve using a third party.
- Give opportunities for the employee to respond formally before decisions are made.
- Allow employees to be accompanied at formal hearings (there is a statutory right for this if the hearing is likely to result in a formal warning or the taking of some other disciplinary action).
- Allow appeals against any formal decisions.

The action from a formal hearing could take the form of a written warning if the case is one of misconduct. In addition to general guidance about employment, there is further guidance on employing nurses by the Nursing and Midwifery Council (NMC, 2011). The NMC recommends that an organisation's internal procedures deal with issues if possible, and this includes disciplinary proceedings. A supportive organisation that can promote continuing professional development to ensure that individuals are fit to practise is preferable to a referral to the NMC. However, there may be cases where the health of the public is compromised, such as a sustained lack of competence. For example:

- Frequent drug/immunisation errors
- Poor judgement
- Lack of knowledge or skill
- Inability to work as part of a team
- Difficulty in communicating with colleagues or people in their care
- Lack of insight into their own lack of competence
- Lack of ability in planning care

As well as the knowledge and skills needed to be fit for practice, a nurse must have good health and character to do their job safely and effectively, and this can be compromised if the nurse has:

- Poor health, such as a neglected and untreated dependence on a substance such as alcohol.
- 'Bad character', such as a serious legal conviction.
- Physical or emotional abuse of people in their care.

Nurses are professionally accountable for their actions, and clearly, reports to the NMC must be made in cases of serious misconduct (NMC, 2008).

What do I do if I feel that I am being bullied?

Bullying behaviour is related to a power imbalance between individuals or groups in relation to another individual or group. It is not confined to children and young people but has become exposed in other areas such as in the workplace (Directgov, 2011). The Anti-Bullying Alliance (ABA, 2011) suggests that organisations form their own specific definition of bullying relevant to the organisation, but that it should include the following general principles:

- Bullying behaviour deliberately causes hurt (either physically or emotionally).
- Bullying behaviour is repetitive (although one-off incidents, such as the posting of an image or the sending of a text that is then forwarded to a group, can quickly become repetitive and spiral into bullying behaviour).
- Bullying behaviour involves an imbalance of power (the person on the receiving end feels as though they cannot defend themselves).

Bullying at work is more specifically about someone trying to intimidate another worker; often this is a manager intimidating an employee, but it may be another co-worker. Bullying is similar to harassment, which is where someone's behaviour is offensive and may include sexual comments or discriminatory language (in relation to race, religion or sexual orientation). Recognising the problem is vital. Many employees do not always recognise that bullying is happening to them, rather like children and young people not understanding appropriate and inappropriate behaviour. Adults often find it difficult to comprehend that they are being bullied and may blame themselves for their own perceived inadequacy rather than face this truth. Feeling threatened at work or not wanting to go to work in the first place should alert individuals to questioning what is happening. Feeling under pressure to conform to the cultural norms of the organisation can have an enormous impact on individual self-esteem and self-confidence. Feeling the physical signs of stress, such as increased anxiety, increased heart rate and blood pressure, frequent headaches and sleeplessness, should be taken seriously.

Examples of bullying (Directgov, 2011)

- Constantly being picked on or criticised
- Being humiliated in front of colleagues
- Regularly unfairly treated
- Physical or verbal abuse

- Being blamed for problems caused by others
- Being given too much work to do, so that you regularly fail in your work
- Regularly threatened with dismissal
- Unfairly passed over for the promotion or denied training opportunities.
- Bullying can be face-to-face or through technology such as email, social networking sites or mobile phones.

Suggested actions

First and foremost, if possible, talk to the relevant person, it may be an unintentional act on their part and you may be able to solve the problem quickly, informally at this level. Being assertive and not aggressive is very important; you are informing the person that you will not tolerate being bullied at any level while maintaining a respectful approach. Further information about assertive skills is included in Chapter 2.

- If the behaviour continues, keep a record of incidents where you feel you have been unfairly treated: record facts, times and your feelings.
- Talk to someone about the issues in confidence. If it is your line manager that is the problem, speak to someone above that.
- Speak to your Human Resources department in confidence. This will then be on record that you have raised concerns.
- Don't allow the situation to go on too long – seek advice early.
- Seek medical help if necessary and record those visits.
- Consider action in relation to grievances – a grievance is a concern or problem that an employee raises with their employer.

What does the law say?

A legal claim about bullying comes under the laws covering harassment and discrimination and if you are forced to resign due to bullying you may be able to make a constructive dismissal claim. For further information on this, visit:

http://www.direct.gov.uk/en/Employment/RedundancyAndLeavingYour-Job/Dismissal/DG_10026696

How do I prioritise my work?

In leading a school health team, acknowledging that you cannot do everything is crucial. Recognition that a mix of skills is valuable and utilising the right skills and knowledge to achieve a common aim is vital. Trusting that members of your team are trained and skilled is your responsibility and allowing them enough freedom to do the job is important. This means having confidence in your team and demonstrating that you trust them. Regular team meetings will allow you to delegate work appropriately and allow opportunities to raise concerns and reinforce the team's goals.

There will be a number of demands on your time and you will need to agree as a team which elements of the work require you personally.

Child protection is a common priority, and for many school nurses across the country this has become the main focus of their work. Although clearly it is important to safeguard children and young people, you need to consider who are the most appropriate people to provide the care package. This may not be the qualified school nurse – there may be another health professional already involved, such as the health visitor – or there may not be a direct health-related problem. Cooperation and negotiation are needed with the management of the school health team to establish real priorities according to the Healthy Child Programme (DH/DfES, 2009), because child protection is only a part of that agenda.

Common priorities include:

- Child protection and child in need (CID)
- Lead professional in the Team Around the Child (TAC)
- Supporting young people in crisis (for example self-harming behaviour, attempted suicide)
- Coordinating immunisation programmes
- Outbreaks of communicable diseases such as TB

It is also necessary to work across the school health service to coordinate work sensibly so that when a problem occurs it can be dealt with. For example, you may have a PSHE or immunisation session booked when a child protection emergency occurs. If the whole service has planned PSHE or immunisation that day, then there will be no cover. However, if the timetable is such that someone else is available then they can step in. It is important to maintain a good relationship with service users at all times, and cancelling booked sessions at short notice is poor practice.

It is important to prioritise time management. If it is not possible to achieve all the work in the hours that you do, then this becomes a management issue. This should be addressed as soon as possible and can also be identified within the appraisal system.

Coping with workload stress
- Manage time effectively.
- Have regular, protected clinical supervision, including child protection supervision.

- Work the hours you are contracted to. If you don't, then the service will never recognise that there is a problem with resources. Equally, don't expect your staff to work more than their contracted hours. This can become a cultural norm and cause friction and stress.
- Audit everything to demonstrate what you are doing. Areas should require this now through IT systems such as RiO. Use this to your advantage to demonstrate a lack of resources if necessary.
- Complete incident forms electronically for any work not covered.
- Be assertive with management and question decisions that affect your workload or changes to your job description.
- Have protected time with family and friends: take time off.

Section 2: Working with children, young people and their families

As a school nurse you will have many skills which will help you deal with all kinds of difficult issues. It is important to remember, however, that each new experience will be unique, and while you are able to draw on previous experiences and knowledge an assessment will help to guide and inform your practice. Asking questions of young people or parents/carers may elicit unexpected responses which may be distasteful, and the listener may not know how to deal with the information. The important thing is to foster relationships in a supportive environment where people feel comfortable sharing things. The school nurse needs also to be a good communicator and must not show extreme emotions such as shock or horror at some of the things they may be told (see Chapter 2). Alongside this, there is the consideration of confidential material: if people share something that leaves either themselves or others at risk, the school nurse cannot guarantee confidentiality. In fact, there is a duty to share this information as part of a child protection process and this gives the message to the person who has disclosed that there is nothing so bad that it cannot be shared with someone. These issues are discussed in Chapters 2 and 6. The school nurse needs to be aware of taking a measured and professional view of the situation: there is no need to overreact. A good understanding of the area guidelines for particular issues is helpful, as is recognition that there may be a number of options which can be planned with the young person. Sometimes it can be helpful for a young person just to be told how brave they have been in disclosing information and how impressive it is that they are coping with the issue. Young people have often dealt with more negative experiences than most people have across a whole lifetime, and they can be told this.

How do I deal with a child that is bullied?

More than ever before in history, children's rights are recognised and acknowledged across the world. It seems incredible that it was not until 1989 that children were given such rights in the Convention on the Rights of the Child (UN, 1989). Children have a human right to an education that is appropriate to their age and which takes place in a safe, positive environment in which to learn (UN, 1989, article 28). The treaty also demands that children learn to respect each other and others' cultures, and to live peacefully (UN, 1989, article 29). Bullying contravenes these basic human rights. The Education and Inspections Act (HM Government, 2006) set out a clear requirement for head teachers to have measures in place in school to deal with bullying. This means that they must have a bullying policy which the school nurse should be encouraged to contribute to. The law also demands that teachers must promote positive behaviour by:

> ... encouraging good behaviour and respect for others on the part of pupils and in particular preventing all forms of bullying among pupils (HM Government, 2006, Part 7 (p. 89)).

The law also requires head teachers to reasonably regulate the behaviour of pupils off school premises, which is a new development in the light of advancing technology. This is very important in today's society, where cyber bullying is becoming a particular problem.

The schools White Paper, *The Importance of Teaching* (DE, 2010) sets out, in Chapter 3, guidance on behaviour and bullying in schools. There is an expectation through this paper that head teachers will establish a 'culture of respect and safety with zero tolerance of bullying' (DE, 2010, p. 32). As we can see from the convention of human rights, this is not a new vision, but we know through groups such as the Anti-Bullying Alliance (ABA) that bullying continues, and that it has become more sophisticated through technology (ABA, 2011). A whole-school approach is necessary, where the ethos is around supporting each other, and young people need to be very clear that bullying is never tolerated by anyone.

The overwhelming evidence from a range of sources and organisations is that bullying is responsible for a range of behaviours including truancy, depression, self-harm and suicide (National Children's Bureau, 2010). In 2006, 2,592 children aged between 11 and 16 were surveyed by the Beatbullying charity, and they found, unsurprisingly, that many children who are bullied avoid school or lessons to get away from the bullies. The case studies within this report make chilling reading, not least because of the attitudes of some schools towards bullying (Beatbullying, 2006). Truancy and avoidance of lessons are clearly going to impact on children and young people's education and therefore, ultimately, their ability to achieve. There have been a range of studies since then which have led the coalition government to focus on behaviour in schools and the powers of teachers to deal with difficult behaviour. Bullying needs to be stopped by using two approaches: prevention and response (NSPCC, 2012).

School nurses have a role to play in both these areas because they have expertise in both preventative work and also in responding to the needs of children and young people. In terms of prevention, the school nurse is in a good position to contribute to individual school behavioural and bullying policies. There are also school nurses working with school staff to raise the self-esteem of children and young people and helping to increase awareness of the importance of developing empathy as well as resilience in children. Because they are also out in the community and part of the child protection agenda, some school nurses are on the local safeguarding boards in relation to bullying. In terms of response, they may be a first point of contact for young people attending school drop-in sessions; they are a safe person to talk to confidentially. They may also be involved with children who are not attending school, and this may be linked directly to bullying behaviour. Co-morbidity is common in young people who are bullied: for example, depression, self-harming behaviour and substance misuse may occur. Young people presenting with these need to be asked about bullying behaviours.

The causes of bullying

Society is aware that bullying is not confined to the school setting, but that it is also present in the community. There have been extreme examples of children assaulting and sometimes murdering other children. Anti-social children run the risk of becoming anti-social adults and the reasons for such behaviours are complex. They include poor parenting, poor early attachments, lack of empathy or foresight, low emotional intelligence, personality disorders, psychiatric disorders, and the possibility that they themselves are being bullied or abused. There is also research which suggests that some bullies have high rather than low self-esteem and that they display behaviours related to arrogance and 'invincibility' (Beatbullying, 2006). As with adults, bullying in children is related to a balance of power and control. A bullied child, for whatever reason, allows someone else to gain control over them, and the psychological reasons for this are multi-faceted.

No one can make you feel inferior without your consent (attributed to Eleanor Roosevelt, n.d.)

Key points to consider on prevention

Children should learn about being a parent in school, and school nurses can contribute to this. Young people need to understand the importance of attachment and emotional development, in particular about emotional intelligence and developing empathy. The 'Roots of Empathy' projects work on this premise and have parents bringing young babies and toddlers into school. The children learn about emotions by understanding the needs of the others. These projects have been shown to have some success in reducing levels of bullying (Gordon, 2009).

Supporting the social development of children is crucial to helping all of them achieve. In this regard, learning respect for others and developing the ability to see another person's perspective is important. The Supporting Emotional Aspects of Learning (SEAL) programmes were introduced in *The Children's Plan* (DCSF, 2007) in both primary and secondary schools. SEAL is:

> a comprehensive, whole-school approach to promoting the social and emotional skills that underpin effective learning, positive behaviour, regular attendance, staff effectiveness and the emotional health and wellbeing of all who learn and work in schools (DCSF, 2007, p. 4).

School nurses across the country contribute to this agenda, providing valuable input into both primary and secondary schools. They can contribute to the overall 'mission statements' of schools, which should be encouraged to embed supporting emotional development across the whole school and not just 'delivering' it through Personal, Health, Social and Economic (PSHE) education.

It is important to consider aspects of resilience. Children who have high levels of resilience are more likely to resist any bullying. Resilience describes the way in which someone is able to cope with changes in their lives – the ability to 'bounce' back from traumatic events. It is about coping strategies. Some children will have low resilience, which could relate to a number of things:

- Low self-esteem/confidence
- Poor self-image or concept
- A feeling of a lack of control
- Introverted or closed personality
- Family background and upbringing
- Inability to develop trusting relationships
- Frequent transitions and life trauma
- Inability to manage feelings effectively
- Anxious/sensitive temperament
- Having an unrealistic view of the world

- Being pessimistic
- Lack of a sense of humour

Having one of these traits does not mean that a child will inevitably be bullied, but possessing a number of these qualities may predispose a child to being vulnerable. The school nurse is in the ideal position to work with children either on a one-to-one basis or in groups. There are a number of resources for schools on building self-esteem and tackling bullying and this is particularly important in the primary schools (NSPCC, 2012). Children moving into secondary school are at increased risk of bullying and transitions for young people can be a particularly problematic time (Children's Workforce Development Council, 2012).

Being 'different' from the norm may pre-dispose a child to bullying and this can take many different forms. Vulnerable groups include those with:

- Learning difficulties
- Mental health problems
- Personality difficulties/disorders
- Special medical needs or a physical disability
- Different sexual orientation from the norm for the environment
- Different race, religion or culture from the norm for that environment

A useful website for further information is: http://youngmindsinschools.org.uk/wellbeing/pupil-wellbeing

Key points to consider on responses to bullying

- School nurses may have children attending drop-ins where disclosures are made about bullying.
- Set clear boundaries around confidentiality. Remember, bullying is a form of abuse.
- Talk to the head teacher. Tackling bullying is a requirement by law. If necessary, you can highlight the problem without breaching confidentiality. Remember, children who disclose want you to do something about it.
- Don't make things worse for the young person; seek advice from your child protection advisor if necessary.
- Listen to the child or young person. Are they at risk of significant harm? Are they suicidal?
- Establish the problem and consider child protection processes.
- Ask the question: 'Are you being bullied?' Tough questions are sometimes very important to assess risk.
- Reassure the young person that this is not their fault.

- Talk to parents if appropriate and be a gatekeeper if necessary to other services, such as Beatbullying, the Anti-Bullying Alliance, Kidscape or CAMHS.
- Use technology positively; give the young person relevant contact details to seek help.
- Evidence has suggested that the use of peer support networks or mentoring systems in schools work well.
- The use of 'Virtual mentors', again using technology, has also been shown to be successful for some young people.
- Liaise with the school; review bullying policies and procedures and consider all options.
- Deal with the bully if appropriate.

Websites to signpost young people to, as of 2012:

- **Anti-Bullying Alliance**: http://www.anti-bullyingalliance.org.uk/
- **Diana Award**: http://diana-award.org.uk/. The Young Anti-Bullying Alliance was formed through a partnership between the Diana Award and the Anti-Bullying Alliance. The Diana Award is in constant touch with more than 10,000 young people in the UK, all of whom have tackled bullying – and continue to do so.
- **Mencap**: http://www.mencap.org.uk/. Dudley's Mencap ME2 group has created an invaluable piece of work based on the bullying of disabled young people.
- **RespectMe**: http://www.respectme.org.uk/. RespectMe is Scotland's anti-bullying service.
- **Stonewall**: http://www.stonewall.org.uk/. Stonewall is the charity that represents lesbians, gay men and bisexuals; a significant part of its work concerns bullying.
- **LGBT History Month**: http://www.lgbthistorymonth.org.uk/; and **Schools Out**: http://www.schools-out.org.uk/.
- **Childnet**: http://www.childnet-int.org/
- **Timebank and T-Mobile**: http://www.txtup.co.uk/. This is a platform that allows young people to share tips and advice with those who may be experiencing bullying by text.
- **Beat Bullying**: http://www.beatbullying.org/. Beat Bullying's CyberMentors programme supports and trains young people to tackle online bullying and to show how technology can support those who have been bullied.

Cyber bullying

It has been argued that today's society has produced three realities or worlds: our internal world, which comprises the inner self; the external world, which comprises the real environmental factors that affect our inner selves; and the digital or virtual world of computers, mobile phones, television, video games and the internet (Byron, 2008). Technology can be a positive asset in terms of using online help groups or cyber mentors, which give young people a platform to talk anonymously if they want to. However, the advance of technology has opened a window of opportunity for bullying online or via text. Social networking sites have created a medium which lends itself to this type of bullying behaviour, creating a 'dark force' of gaining control over someone else's life which is very difficult to monitor (Byron, 2008).

A study done by EU Kids Online between 2009 and 2011 on 25,142 9–16-year-olds in 25 countries showed that Internet use in this age group is increasing and that on average children spend 88 minutes per day online either via mobile or computer (EU Kids Online, 2011). This study shows the complex nature of bullying behaviour in young people. Half of those who bully online are likely to also bully face-to-face and also, interestingly, among those who have been bullied online, nearly half have also bullied someone else (EU Kids Online, 2011). Access to the Internet is increasing through mobile phones and handheld devices, and it should be acknowledged that there are some positives about the access to information. Social networking sites allow young people to communicate and have fun, but many users of these sites are under age (9–12-year-olds), including 20% on Facebook and 38% using social networking sites overall (EU Kids Online, 2011). Understanding of privacy and disclosure is really important for young people and there have been cases of young people posting pictures of themselves naked or in compromising positions without the full understanding that these pictures may be fully accessed and that they cannot be erased (see Case study 3.3).

The law requires head teachers to extend their care to their pupils beyond the school gates, but this is very difficult to achieve given the increasing access to networking sites. Monitoring young people's behaviour requires cooperation from parents, but there are many reasons why parents do not engage with the protection of their children. Early warnings to children who grow up using computers are important, along with the skills to resist the bully, but children will often ignore advice about using the Internet (EU Kids Online, 2011).

There have also been a number of cases of young people running away from home to meet people who they have met online. This raises concerns about sexual exploitation and has become commonly known as grooming (see Case study 3.4).

Case study 3.3

Amy, aged 9, visited her friend Chelsea at home after school. Chelsea was a single child who spent a lot of time in her bedroom alone on her computer. Amy went home really upset as she said that Chelsea was talking to someone online and then took her knickers down and was touching herself. She then took a pen and inserted the pen into her vagina. Chelsea said that it was OK and not to tell anyone and that she knew how to erase the history from her computer. We can only guess that the person online had taught her how to do this. Amy was so upset that she thought about going to the policeman next door, but instead told her mum when she got home. Her mum phoned Chelsea's mum who refused to believe it and said it was a malicious story made up by Amy. She then spoke to the head teacher at school who said that it was a community issue and nothing to do with him. Amy's mum was really concerned about upsetting Chelsea's mum and did not know what to do next. The school nurse (a) advised Chelsea's mum to reported it to the police, (b) reported it to the online protection team and (c) spoke to the duty officer at children's social care.

Case study 3.4

A 14-year-old girl was reported missing by her family. She had been groomed online by a 42-year-old man who had taken her away to a hotel. When she was found she was adamant that he loved her and she loved him. She was reluctant to give a police statement and refused any sexual health services. These men are very clever at choosing vulnerable young girls to prey on and the girls are so keen for affection that they seem blind to the reality. Education has to play a key role in boosting self-esteem. The man was arrested and charged and is currently serving a prison sentence.

How do I deal with young victims who do not know that they are being abused?

Exploitative behaviour, including both the face-to-face and online approaches of sexual predators, is a worrying problem for young people. The lack of awareness or acknowledgement of young people that they are being abused is clearly portrayed both in real life case studies described by practitioners and in fictional soap operas such as *EastEnders*. Soap operas are a valuable way of informing young people of real-life dangers because they are watched by millions of teenagers. Soaps can be used effectively to discuss sensitive issues as they enable discussion of a third party which 'one step removes' potentially personal topics (see Protective Behaviours, 2012). They are (generally speaking) done well, with the odd exception.

In 2011 *EastEnders* ran a chilling story of sexual exploitation of a main character (Whitney). The pattern of behaviour is the befriending of a young person by an older man who buys the affection of the vulnerable young person by giving presents, listening to their problems and helping them make decisions about their lives. The perpetrator gradually isolates the young person from their friends and family, setting themselves up as the only one that truly understands, cares or loves them. Once this trusting relationship is developed, the sexual favours can be introduced, first with the perpetrator and then later for his friends or clients. Thus he in effect becomes a pimp and makes money from the sexual encounters. The victim is generally so isolated by this stage that they either still believe that they are loved and are in love or are too scared to get out of the situation. Even more worrying is when the whole family becomes involved in the situation (Case study 3.5). Tackling this problem will clearly involve a multi-agency approach, which also involves society as a whole taking social responsibility for the safety of children and young people.

Case study 3.5

Cassie was 14 years old and was found guilty of shoplifting and given a community warning. The police officer dealing with her case asked me to see her as she was smoking and keen to give up. He was also concerned that she might be sexually active and asked me to discuss this with her to make sure she was 'safe' from the risk of pregnancy or sexually transmitted infections. I met Cassie and was struck by how compliant and helpful she was. Sometimes young people are particularly keen to help, and although this can be seen as a positive trait it may also be indicative of someone who has been manipulated to be compliant.

She was pleasant and chatty and we completed a health assessment. There was a readiness to try to stop smoking. During the time spent together we started to discuss relationships and she told me that she had a boyfriend, Jonny. She was obviously very keen on him and had in fact run away from school on a couple of occasions to be with him. He was 20 years old, which immediately caused concerns as the age difference at this time is significant. Her mum had reported her missing and children's social care did call an SOS (Signs of Safety) meeting to formulate a multi-professional approach to keeping Cassie safe.

Cassie's father had sexually abused her when she was younger and when found guilty had been sent to prison. Her mum, who had not known she was being abused, has terrible feelings of guilt. This has resulted in her having difficulty in imposing boundaries on Cassie, as she does not want to upset her. However, the consequence of this is that Cassie is pushing the boundaries too far and into potentially hazardous situations.

We then received information that Jonny was a settled traveller, but had stolen from his family and had been made homeless. He had then been housed in supported lodgings, outside the local area.

Cassie had very low self-esteem and her face lit up when she showed me the new coat she was wearing, which Jonny had given her. She also said that he had promised her a handbag. She was delighted to be shown such affection and took this to mean that he was really 'in love' with her. I felt uncomfortable that he was showering her with gifts and noted early warning signals of possible grooming. Jonny was now being welcomed into the family home, as her mum reasoned that at least she would know she was safe. Cassie told me that her mum really liked him and he had bought her mum a bottle of wine. It could be that he was kind and generous, but both Cassie and her mum were very vulnerable to being taken advantage of. People who behave like Jonny are usually charming, manipulative and very plausible. On the follow up SOS meeting I asked Cassie's mum who was looking after her younger two girls. She said that she had left them at home with Jonny babysitting. He had made himself invaluable to the whole family.

It was really difficult to know how to proceed, but I discussed sexual health with Cassie, did some work on self-esteem and as delicately as possible gave her some scenarios and pitfalls to be aware of with young men. I could tell that she registered what I was saying, and although she said that nothing like that had happened to her I could tell she was relating some of it to her own situation. I talked about the risks to her mum, who found it difficult as she felt that since he had been round more, at least she was not running away.

Her mum is trying to do the right thing, but is not sure what that is. A parenting worker has been involved to help her to enforce boundaries. I have accompanied Cassie to the sexual health clinic to take appropriate care. She is working on smoking cessation. I have given her contact details for myself and other services should she find herself in a situation where she may need to speak to someone.

It is really hard because all you can do is give the information and hope that the young person has enough self-esteem to be able to say no and to seek help before things get out of hand. It is rarely completely obvious what is happening and is often more subtle. Even though everyone involved in her case was concerned that she was being groomed and exploited, there was never enough evidence to act. Subsequently, services have had to withdraw and hope that this young girl stays safe. The men who do the grooming choose the girls and families who have low self-esteem and are vulnerable. They shower them with affection and gifts, masking their real intent. They build up trust with charm and generosity and then start to abuse the girls for self-gratification.

These girls and families crave positive attention, and because it has often been lacking are not good at judging between good and bad.

The parenting worker is still working with the family and we hope we have at least given the family the 'tools' to recognise when things are not quite right and the confidence to act accordingly.

The role of the school nurse

- Be alert to the problem
- Refer to social care
- Talk to the school: remember, as with bullying, head teachers are required to address problems outside the school gates
- Liaise with police and other professionals: report behaviour
- Refer to child exploitation and online protection (CEOP)
- Early warnings to children and young people
- Inform parents regularly about the problem at any parents groups where there is an opportunity to do so
- Make sure parents know what their child is viewing online
- Build self-esteem in children and be aware of bullying in school
- Be aware of co-morbidity, such as substance misuse, self-harm and depression
- Understand vulnerability

For further information visit:

- **Child Exploitation and Online Protection**: http://www.ceop.police.uk/
- **Family Online Safety Institute**: http://www.fosi.org/
- **The Anna Freud Institute**: http://www.annafreud.org/corc.htm

How do I deal with children and young people who self-harm?

Closely linked to bullying is self-harming behaviour. Deliberate self-harm covers a range of behaviours, from hair pulling, head banging and cutting to suicide. There remains a lack of full understanding about why people self-harm, but the quote below is a commonly expressed explanation by those who self-injure:

> When I cut myself I feel so much better, all the little things that might have been annoying me suddenly seem so trivial because I'm concentrating on the pain. I'm not a person who can scream and shout so this is my only outlet. It's all done very logically. (*Richey Edwards of the rock group Manic Street Preachers, who went missing in 1995. He is thought to have committed suicide but his body has never been found.*)

Young people who self-harm do so for a range of reasons and the role of the school nurse is similar to that of supporting young people who have been bullied. Co-morbidities with self-harm are common, often aligned with substance misuse, depression, anxiety disorders or emerging personality disorder (Mind, 2012). As well as this, there is often a history of abuse. With many issues that relate to supporting mental health and wellbeing, the key to successful therapeutic intervention is the trust that the young person has in the individual that they approach. In reality, this could be anyone, including teachers, nurses, friends, parents, youth workers or counsellors. Dealing with distressing information can often cause real anxiety for individuals and a fear that one is not trained to deal with some issues. Therefore it is vital to have systems in place that allow a free flow of information in order to best support a young person's needs.

Dr Dickon Bevington, a child psychiatrist with the Anna Freud Centre, suggests that to maximise the most effective treatments for young people a key worker model should be adopted, with the direct care and intervention done by one person and other professionals working around that key worker (Bevington, 2012). He claims that too often, so many people become involved in trying to help that the real needs of the young person become lost. A school nurse would seem an ideal person as they are the only health professional directly involved with school age children that they can access directly and confidentially. Therefore, school nurses need to align themselves with Child and Adolescent Mental Health Services (CAMHS), and indeed they are doing so in many areas.

Many school nurses across the country are working at Tier 1 and Tier 2 mental health support. It is important to have clinical support when working with these children and clinical supervision with CAMHS is essential for advice and referrals. Many areas now have these links to CAMHS and school nurses report that they are able to help more effectively and confidently when they have this support. With increasing referrals to CAMHS the thresholds have changed, meaning that only the most serious cases are taken by CAMHS. This means that more work is done at Tier 1 and Tier 2.

The structure of CAMHS

- **Tier 1: Universal – generic and primary services (including prevention)**
  Support at this level is done by practitioners who are not mental health specialists working in universal services; this includes GPs, health visitors, school nurses, teachers, social workers, youth justice workers and voluntary agencies. Practitioners will be able to offer general advice and treatment for less severe problems, contribute towards mental health promotion, identify problems early in their development, and refer to more specialist services.

- **Tier 2: Targeted input (prevention – intervention) locality-based CAMHS across agencies**
  This tier can include primary mental health workers, psychologists and counsellors working in GP practices, paediatric clinics, schools and youth services. With a stretched CAMHS it also increasingly is a level at which school nurses are working. Practitioners offer consultation to families and other practitioners; outreach to identify severe or complex needs which require more specialist interventions; and assessment (which may lead to treatment at a different tier).

- **Tier 3: Specialist services (locality-based CAMHS specialists)**
  This is usually a multidisciplinary team or service working in a community mental health clinic or child psychiatry outpatient service, providing a specialised service for children and young people with more severe, complex and persistent disorders. Team members are likely to include child and adolescent psychiatrists, social workers, clinical psychologists, community psychiatric nurses, child psychotherapists, occupational therapists, and art, music and drama therapists.

- **Tier 4: Specialised services (client-specific)**
  These are essential tertiary level services for children and young people with the most serious problems; such services may be day units, highly-specialised outpatient teams and inpatient units. These can include secure forensic adolescent units, eating disorders units, specialist neuro-psychiatric teams, and other specialist teams (for children who have been sexually abused, for example), usually serving more than one district or region.

School nurses are not trained counsellors but have the communication skills to listen to children and young people and recognise when they need more expert help (see Chapter 2). Anyone who is likely to encounter young people who self-harm needs training in assessing risk. The National Institute for Health and Clinical Excellence (NICE) guidelines recommend the use of the Australian mental health triage scale when assessing someone who has self-harmed (NICE, 2004).

As with child protection guidance, if a child or young person is at risk of immediate significant harm or they are likely to harm someone else, then this will require immediate action.

The key guiding principles for primary care from NICE are:

- Assess immediate risk of physical harm – refer to hospital if necessary/call an ambulance/police.
- Consider the mental health and emotional state of the young person – identify the main demographic and clinical features and psychological characteristics, such as depression, hopelessness or ongoing suicidal tendencies.
- Treat people with respect, care and privacy.
- Show compassion and understanding.
- Assessment needs to include an exploration of the individual's feelings and thoughts about the self-harming behaviour.
- Explore other coping strategies.
- Involve young people in any decisions that are made about their care.
- A psychosocial assessment should be made – this includes background, family, friends, ambitions etc.
- Support the family or friends if appropriate.
- Effective collaboration with other services.
- Staff should have regular clinical supervision.
- Consider issues around consent and mental capacity.
- Harm minimisation strategies: reduce the risks for young people if they continue to self-harm; clean equipment for example.

The skills required for this work are discussed further in Chapter 2.

What about children and young people who are abusing substances?

The school nurse can contribute to this agenda by working closely with other agencies involved in this issue, such as drugs actions teams, youth workers, schools and the police. In many areas, the multi-agency drop-ins include people from these agencies, and therefore this is the most effective way to address substance misuse among young people. Working in cooperation with the police and youth services to provide education for both children and parents is also important, and having a health input into these areas is crucial. Many young people have their first sexual experience under the influence of alcohol and may access the school nurse following this for sexual health advice. This is a good opportunity to discuss health promotion and risk-taking behaviour with young people. From a child and adolescent development perspective, evidence suggests that there are physical reasons for risk-taking behaviour: the frontal cortex, responsible for rational thought and judgement is developing during adolescence and is the last part of the brain to become 'hard wired' (Giedd, 2009). Social developmental theorists also suggest that adolescence is a time of gaining independence and emancipation from parents, which can make the teenage years a troublesome time (Herbert, 2003).

It seems almost accepted that many teenagers will go through a time of rebellion, and some teenagers will drink alcohol through this period of transition – certainly the media portrayal of young people offers this perception. There is an annual survey done on young people's drinking and smoking habits in participating schools, which in fact reported that alcohol consumption has gone down in young people (NHS Information Centre, 2010). However, the survey also shows that those who are drinking, are drinking more.

When the use of substances such as alcohol is becoming problematic, this needs to be recognised. This may be related to developing an addiction, which can be difficult to clearly define as clients and professionals may have a different view of what it means. It could be described as an activity that becomes a pre-occupation or a craving and there seems to be general agreement that addiction is about becoming dependent and losing control over one's actions (WHO, 2012). With young people, developing a dependency when the brain is at a crucial stage of development may have serious long-term consequences on their ability to lead a healthy, useful life. The latest research across the world suggests that the key substances that young people use are alcohol, cannabis and ecstasy, and there are few young people who become involved in other drugs such as heroin (UN, 2011). The Healthy Child Programme acknowledges this agenda and school nurses can contribute through PSHE education and providing accessible services for young people (DCSF/DH, 2009).

How do I reach disadvantaged or marginalised groups?

A challenge for all professionals working with children and young people is accessing those who fall outside the 'existing frameworks of service provision' (Home Office, 2004, p. 3). These can be defined in three main groups:

■ Minority groups who are marginalised, disadvantaged or socially excluded, for example gypsies and travellers or asylum seekers.

■ Those who are 'invisible' or unable to articulate their needs, such as young carers, those with mental health problems or those who fall just outside the thresholds for intervention.

■ Those who are unwilling to engage with service providers. These young people may include those who are disaffected or suspicious of professionals for a range of reasons: they may be substance users, have been in care, have had a negative previous experience of professionals or be involved in crime. They may also be those who are being groomed.

If young people are in school, then there is an increased chance that the school nurse will be able to offer a health service. If they are not, it becomes much more difficult. However, school nurses have a responsibility to school-age children, whether they are in school or not. This needs to be a consideration when thinking about the most appropriate people to engage young people.

Key considerations:

■ Networking – be aware of anyone who works with marginalised or vulnerable populations either professionally or voluntarily in your area:
  – Outreach education services
  – Specialised health visitors or school nurses liaising with vulnerable groups
  – Drugs and alcohol teams
  – Youth services
  – Social services
  – Young carers
  – Connexions
  – Educational Welfare Office
  – Youth Offending Service
  – Looked after children's nurses
■ Be clear about your role; are you the most appropriate person in the situation or does someone else have more appropriate skills or knowledge?
■ Are there community liaison individuals who will speak for the community to develop better understanding?
■ Consider child protection and the law and maintain a professional approach – this can be particularly difficult, but ethical implications and accountability should be a consideration. Think about the best interests of the child or young person.

- Develop understanding of the specific culture or subculture that you are dealing with.
- Ask young people what they want.
- Assess risk to yourself and others when engaging with individuals or groups.
- Develop good communication skills in order to build trust.
- Be clear about assessing need; it is important to have the resources to address any identified need before you start.

How do I respond to looked after children's needs?

> ... when I was in foster care, I felt that no one was listening to me. At the reviews, there would be six or seven adults and me. It is not easy to be honest in that situation. I always felt that being in care was my fault and I was being blamed for it by the professionals. They need to listen more to me and my needs. I was placed in a boys' school which I hated and this is why I failed my GCSEs. I understand that the social workers are doing their job but it is not my fault I was in care...'. (A 20-year-old who had been in looked after care).

Some areas have designated looked after children's nurses. They are specialist nurses who promote the health and wellbeing of children in care. They work closely with school nurses and others to offer a holistic approach to the health and social needs of children and young people. Health assessments can be done in school if appropriate or in the home if necessary. As school nurses are already going into school, they are sensible people to assess health needs and are also well placed to promote health. A school drop-in provides a good opportunity to see young people which does not stigmatise them or alienate them further from the rest of the school population. However, the wishes of the child or young person need be acknowledged, and some may not want a visit in school as this may draw unwanted attention to them; a home visit may be more appropriate. As the above quote suggests, listening to children in care is vital and acting as an advocate important.

There are statutory requirements to monitor the health of looked after children and well-documented poor health, social and educational outcomes for these children. In 2010, NICE and the Social Care Institute for Excellence (SCIE) produced guidelines for improving the quality of life for looked after children (NICE/SCIE, 2010). The guidance recommends that it is implemented alongside: *Statutory Guidance on Promoting the Health and Well-being of Looked After Children* (DCSF/DH, 2009) and *The Children Act 1989 Guidance and Regulations Volume 2: Care Planning, Placement and Case Review* (HM Government, 2010).

The recommendations in the NICE/SCIE guidelines are:

■ Put the voices of children, young people and their families at the heart of service design and delivery.
■ Deliver services that are tailored to the individual and diverse needs of children and young people by ensuring effective joint commissioning and integrated professional working.
■ Develop services that address health and wellbeing and promote high-quality care.
■ Encourage warm and caring relationships between child and carer that nurture attachment and create a sense of belonging so that the child or young person feels safe, valued and protected
■ Help children and young people to develop a strong sense of personal identity and maintain the cultural and religious beliefs they choose.
■ Ensure young people are prepared for and supported in their transition to adulthood.
■ Support the child or young person to participate in the wider network of peer, school and community activities to help build resilience and a sense of belonging.
■ Ensure children and young people have a stable experience of education that encourages high aspiration and supports them in achieving their potential.

Conclusions

The potential role of the school nurse seems immense. Recognition that practitioners cannot work in isolation is key; the school nurse service varies across the country and there are different needs in different areas, all of which needs to be taken into consideration. Trying to standardise the role is problematic and the skill you need as a school nurse team leader is to be able to assess this need and prioritise the input needed. As new political agendas arise around children and young people, the school nurse needs to be flexible in order to meet the needs of children and young people in their specific area. With cuts to children's services it may be that the role of the SN will increase as one of the few practitioners still in post to address some of these needs. This will place inevitable strain on the service, and skill mix may provide the answer. However, the key is to put the needs of children at the centre of the services and ensure that the most suitable person is meeting their needs. This will mean new ways of working across professional boundaries and this may be crucial to meeting young people's needs in a time of public service cuts. This is not a new way of thinking – many barriers have prevented this model working in the past – but it remains imperative that different ways of working are explored and developed.

References

ACAS (2009) *Disciplinary and Grievance Procedures*, Stationery Office, London.

Anti-Bullying Alliance (2012) *What is Bullying?* Available at http://www.abatoolsfor-schools.org.uk/what_is_bullying/what_is_bullying.aspx (accessed 19 March 2012).

Beatbullying (2006) *Shaping Behaviour, Changing Attitudes*. Available at http://www.beatbullying.org/index.html (accessed 15 March 2011).

Belbin, M. (1981) *Management Teams*. Heinemann, London.

Bevington, D. (2012) *AMBIT: A New Approach to Helping Troubled Young People*. Available at http://www.annafreud.org/pages/ambit.html (accessed 14 January 2012).

Business Balls (2011) *Tuckman, forming, storming, norming, performing model*. ONLINE from: http://www.businessballs.com/tuckmanformingstormingnormingperforming.htm Accessed Dec 29th 2011.

Byron, T. (2008) *Safer Children in a Digital World*. DCSF Publications, London.

Children's Workforce Development Council [CWDC] (2012) *Supporting Transitions*. Available at http://www.cwdcouncil.org.uk/young-peoples-workforce/skills-development-framework-online/sdf/level-3/supporting-transitions (accessed 13 January 2012).

Costa, P. T. Jr and McCrae, R. R. (1992) *Revised NEO Personality Inventory (NEO-PI-R) and NEO Five-Factor Inventory (NEO-FFI) Manual*. Psychological Assessment Resources, Odessa, FL.

Department for Children, Schools and Families (2007) *The Children's Plan*. DCSF, London.

Department for Children, Schools and Families/Department of Health (2009) *Statutory Guidance on Promoting the Health and Well-being of Looked After Children*. DCSF/DH, London.

Department for Education (2010) *The Importance of Teaching*. DE, London.

Department of Health/Department for Children, Schools and Families (2009) *The Healthy Child Programme from 5 to 19*. DH/DCSF, London.

DirectGov (2011) *Bullying in the Workplace*. Available at http://www.direct.gov.uk/en/Employment/ResolvingWorkplaceDisputes/DiscriminationAtWork/DG_10026670 (accessed 12 January 2012).

EU Kids Online (2011) *EU Kids Online Report September 2011*. Available at http://www2.lse.ac.uk/media@lse/research/EUKidsOnline/Home.aspx (accessed 14 January 2012).

Giedd, J. (2009) *The Teen Brain: Primed to Learn, Primed to Take Risks*. Available at http://www.dana.org/news/cerebrum/detail.aspx?id=19620 (accessed 24 October 2011).

Gordon, M. (2009) *Roots of Empathy*. The Experiment, New York.

Herbert, M. (2003) *Typical and Atypical Development: From Conception to Adolescence.* Blackwell, Oxford.

HM Government (2006) *Education and Inspections Act.* HM Government, London.

HM Government (2010). *The Children Act 1989 Guidance and Regulations Volume 2: Care Planning, Placement and Case Review.* HM Government, London.

Home Office (2004*) Delivering Services to Hard to Reach Families in on Track Areas: Definitions, Consultation and Needs Assessment.* Home Office, Research, Development and Statistics Directorate, London.

Lewin, K. (1951) *Field Theory in Social Science; Selected Theoretical Papers.* Harper & Row, New York.

MBTI (2012) *The Myers Briggs Foundation.* Available at http://www.myersbriggs.org/ (accessed 13 January 2012).

Mind (2012) *Understanding Self-harm.* Available at http://www.mind.org.uk/help/diagnoses_and_conditions/self-harm (accessed 14 January 2012).

National Children's Bureau [NCB] (2010) *Bullying. Highlight No 261* NCB, London.

NHS Information Centre (2010) *Smoking, Drinking and Drug Use Among Young People in England.* NHS Information Centre, London.

NICE (2004) *Self-harm: the Short-term Physical and Psychological Management and Secondary Prevention of Self-harm in Primary and Secondary Care.* NICE, London.

NICE/SCIE (2010) *Looked After Children and Young People.* NICE, London.

Nursing and Midwifery Council [NMC] (2008) *The Code. Standards of Conduct, Performance and Ethics for Nurses and Midwives.* NMC, London.

NMC (2011) *Advice and Information for Employers of Nurses and Midwives.* NMC, London.

NSPCC (2012) *Bullying: Resources for Schools and Teachers on Bullying* Available at http://www.nspcc.org.uk/Inform/resourcesforteachers/classroomresources/bullying_wda55551.html (accessed 13 January 2012).

Protective Behaviours (2012) Available at http://www.protectivebehaviours.co.uk/ (accessed 19 March 2012).

United Nations (1989) *The Convention on the Rights of the Child.* UN.

United Nations (2011) *World Drug Report 2011.* United Nations Office on Drugs and Crime.

World Health Organization [WHO] (2012) *Lexicon of Alcohol and Drug Terms Published by the World Health Organization.* Available at http://www.who.int/substance_abuse/terminology/who_lexicon/en/ (accessed 14 January 2012).

CHAPTER 4

Child protection

Kate Potter and Jane Wright

Key themes in this chapter:

- What is the school nurse role in child protection?
- What are the latest recommendations for safeguarding children and young people?
- Examples of real life cases and their outcomes
- Useful resources

Introduction

Child protection has become an increasingly significant part of the role of the school nurse. This aspect of working with children can be challenging and at times stressful, and it is important that all practitioners within school nursing teams are aware of their responsibilities. Regular updates on safeguarding and child protection should occur in the practice setting in a multi-agency arena, and awareness of national and local protocols is mandatory for everyone. This chapter is intended as an overview of the child protection process and a clarification of the terms currently in use and should be used in conjunction with practice guidelines. It includes a series of real-life case studies from school nurses working in different areas of the UK. The case studies illustrate the role of the school nurse in the child protection process. Examples from all of the categories of abuse will be given and all names have been changed to ensure confidentiality in line with NMC guidelines (NMC, 2008).

The legislation, policy and procedures for the protection of children in the UK have developed in response to critical cases over more than a century. In the last ten years there have been separate policies developed across the three devolved countries: Scotland, Northern Ireland and Wales. The systems in place across all four countries remain very similar, with the focus on developing systems which are right for the child (Stafford *et al.*, 2010). In June 2010, Eileen Munro was asked to review child protection in England. She noted a significant rise in referrals to social care between 2008/2009 and 2009/2010 (Munro, 2011). Perhaps this increase was understandable, given the case of Peter Connelly and Lord Laming's Review of Safeguarding in 2009 (Laming, 2009). She also highlighted the processes that have developed with regard to IT (form filling, rules and procedures and targets), which she claims limit the actual time that is spent with children and their families. This time with families, it is claimed, is vital to build relationships and assess parenting capacity.

Munro gives clear recommendations which impact directly on the work of the school nurse. Her final report is sub-titled 'a child centred system', and all school nurses are in the position to be developing services which hear the 'voice of the child' (Office for Standards in Education [Ofsted], 2011). She also recognises that early intervention is key in the prevention of many cases of abuse. This is supported by the growing belief that child protection is a public health issue and governments should recognise it as such (Barlow and Calam, 2011).

Local policies and protocols for child protection are now kept on the intranet systems of NHS trusts to enable timely updates without the need to produce a hard copy. This ensures that all are working to the most current guidance. Any amendments are usually cascaded via an email to all staff, whose responsibility is then to be familiar with any changes. All staff should receive regular multi-agency training at levels dependent on their responsibility (Royal College of Paediatrics and Child Health [RCPCH], 2010). The named nurse for child protection is also an invaluable resource for advice and guidance, and it is good practice to contact them as soon as you have concerns around a child and their family. Clinical supervision for child protection is also a requirement (Munro, 2008). This provides a safe opportunity to reflect on the case and identify the best way forward to achieve the safety and best outcomes for the child and, hopefully, their family. The model for this supervision is often a group of practitioners facilitated by a specialist practitioner in child protection. This is a crucial opportunity to learn from the practice of more experienced practitioners.

At this point it is important to acknowledge the emotional burden of working with the children who are suffering abuse or neglect, or who are exposed to other risks of significant harm. With the increasing size of school nurse caseloads and more child protection work, the amount of time required to support children who are at risk of harm, write reports, and attend case conferences and core groups is significant (Ford, 2009). School nurses are often working with families with extremely complex needs and situations, which can be very distressing. Practitioners must ensure that they have the required support for their own wellbeing.

Support frameworks

- Newly-employed and newly-qualified staff should have a programme of preceptorship (see Chapter 2).
- Regular meetings with the school health team.
- Clinical supervision.
- Immediate access to the named nurse for child protection, and also availability for less urgent concerns.
- Access to social care child protection team for informal telephone advice.

The importance of good interagency working is fundamental to a system which works to protect children and support families (DE, 2010). Practitioners need to understand their own roles and responsibilities, and they can then work towards the key principles of successful interprofessional working. These are:

- A clear understanding of the roles of other professionals.
- Effective communication between professionals.
- Respect for other professionals.

Practitioners working in school health teams may have gained experience of integrated working in child protection when working with Common Assessment Frameworks (CAF), as members of a Team Around a Child (TAC) or have taken the lead professional role. There is good evidence that for families, the experience of CAFs and TACs improves outcomes for families and also improves inter-agency working (DE, 2010). It has been continuously illustrated that sharing information across agencies is the key to ensuring that safe and informed decisions are made around protecting children (Laming, 2009; Munro, 2011). Health professionals are often concerned about issues of confidentiality, and for school nurses there are issues around the betrayal of the trust of the child. The main principles to remember are that the safety of the child or vulnerable adult is paramount. The decision for what information should be shared must be made on a 'need to know' basis. There are clear guidelines on information sharing for all practitioners (HM Government, 2008a) (see Chapters 3 and 6).

The referral system for 'children at risk of harm', rather than those in need, should be different. Practitioners must be clear and confident of where and how to refer. They also need to be able to clearly articulate their concerns and identify the key factors which are indicating that the child is at risk of or is suffering significant harm. This is the point where discussion with the named nurse for child protection can help clarify concerns. They work on a rota system, so there should always be someone to ask for advice.

Social workers are formally obliged to carry out a Section 47 enquiry when there is 'reasonable cause to suspect' that a child is, or is likely to suffer 'significant harm' (DE, 2010). The result of this enquiry is likely to be a convening of an initial Child Protection Case Conference.

General checklist for child protection conferences

- Collate all appropriate information about the child and family from your and your service's involvement with the child. This should include all aspects of their engagement with health services. It is appropriate to speak to other professionals who may be currently, or have in the past been, involved with the family. This would include health visitors, GPs, speech therapists, voluntary agencies and schools.
- Arrange to see child/children for a health assessment prior to attending an initial child protection case conference, preferably on a home visit following a risk assessment. This is a good opportunity to meet the family in their own environment and establish a relationship.
- Write a report using the locally approved template. This should also use the assessment triangle (CAF) to ensure that all factors for the child/children are taken into consideration. It is important to include any positive aspects, such as a supportive extended family nearby. There is also an expectation that you are able to provide an informed and critical approach to the report using your knowledge of child development, and that you can identify specific risks of harm in specific situations, for instance domestic violence.
- Share the report with the family to ensure that there are no surprises at the case conference. Even unpalatable information is often received by the clients in an accepting way, as they are often very aware of the basis of concerns which have been raised by professionals. Families often have trust in health professionals.
- Send the report, in advance, to the child protection office in time to be included in a pack of reports for presentation at the conference.
- Attend the conference. Local policy may vary, but often a named nurse for child protection will attend initial conferences too.
- The conference will highlight areas of work required and identify who is responsible for each element, and a plan of work will be agreed.
- Decisions around whether the child/children should be subject to a child protection plan can be contentious. It is important that you are able to be clear about your opinion and also that you ensure that if you do not agree with the decision that this is recorded in the minutes of the conference.

- Your role will continue as part of a child protection plan. You will be part of the multiprofessional core group who will meet regularly to monitor progress and the health and wellbeing of the child/children. You should be sure that any responsibilities that you undertake in this role are part of your remit as a school nurse and are focused on the health and emotional wellbeing of the child or young person. You may also want to consider here the most appropriate person for this role. A health visitor may be also involved, for example, or you may have a very experienced staff nurse who is capable of taking on the case. The School Nurse Development Programme (DH, 2012) recommends that school nurses as leaders should be aware of the skills of all their team members.
- Write review conference report using the local child protection paperwork agreed through the safeguarding boards.

A case conference can be a daunting experience for staff and clients, and although evidence is explored, judgements do have to be made and this can feel very uncomfortable. It is important to keep the child in the centre of the picture and imagine what it is like to be that child – this can help to focus on what is needed to ensure the best possible outcomes. Also, we do not work in isolation and colleagues from partner agencies all contribute to improving the life chances for children and young people to help them achieve (Trodd and Chivers, 2011).

The threshold for cases changing from 'children in need' to 'child protection' is quite high. It can be difficult to understand why some do and some do not, and as professionals we need to be confident about asking for clarification from children's social care and be prepared to challenge if necessary. It can sometimes be appropriate to speak to the independent chair of the conference if there is concern about the decision. For newly-qualified staff this may seem quite daunting, but we have to 'work in the best interest of the child'. 'As a professional, you are personally accountable for actions and omissions in your practice and must always be able to justify your decisions' (NMC, 2008). It is also important to continue to support and monitor families when it is decided that at this point they do not require a child protection plan, especially where you have some concerns.

At the present time neglect is the most common reason for children to be subject to a child protection plan. In March 2010 there were 20,481 children recorded in this category in the UK (NSPCC, 2011). Awareness of neglect and also the effect it has on the future development of children has continued to increase over the last twenty years (Daniel *et al.*, 2011). Deciding thresholds for referral and also for assessing risk of significant harm is often the most difficult in this category. Recording of all concerns and for school nurses focusing on the impact on health and emotional wellbeing is crucial.

The following case studies focus on particular areas of abuse. It is helpful to revisit the clear definitions within *Working Together* (DH, 2010) and consider why in these cases children were suffering or likely to suffer significant harm under the suggested category. Each of the case studies highlights some key issues raised within the case and speculates on what early interventions may have helped the situation. The drive within *the Healthy Child Programme from Pregnancy to Five* and *The Healthy Child Programme from 5–19* (DH/DCSF 2009) is to intervene early in order to improve outcomes for children in need. This means considering how to work with parents and form partnerships across disciplines to promote the health and wellbeing of families.

Case study 4.1: Neglect

Family history

Amy was 10 years old at the time of referral and is an only child. She lives with her father (Jon) who was unemployed and is an alcoholic. Amy's mother had died two years before of breast cancer. Jon has a sister, Hannah, who lives nearby but who works full time and has three children of her own. Amy's maternal grandparents live some distance away and her paternal grandparents had both died since the death of Amy's mother. The family are Christians who attended church regularly until the death of Amy's mother; since then, attendance has been reduced to occasional visits. It transpires that this was often because Jon was finding it difficult to get up in the mornings to go to church.

The child protection issue

Amy had disclosed to a teacher that she was often waiting in the car in a car park for her father (Jon) while he was drinking in the local pub. When concerns were first raised over this disclosure the child protection thresholds were not met. New concerns were raised shortly afterwards, however, by the school, due to visible head lice on Amy's head. There were also concerns about Amy's schoolwork and attitude in class, which had gradually deteriorated since her mother had died. Amy had started school as a lively and enthusiastic student who made friends easily, but she had become withdrawn and anxious and lacked concentration, often falling asleep in class. There had also been a social care referral due to Jon's persistent lateness in picking her up from school.

School nurse involvement

The school nurse observed Amy from a distance in the classroom. Head lice were visible from several feet away. She was also observed to be quiet and withdrawn, and other children were avoiding sitting with her. It was important not to single her out in front of her peers, so the school nurse spoke to Jon, who agreed to accept help. The school nurse did a home visit with the 'bug busting kit'. This involves careful combing of wet hair with a fine-toothed comb. Head lice were present at all stages of their development and the hair was matted with blood. There had been hair loss around the neck line, which indicated that head lice had been present for a long time.

Following a discussion with Jon, a referral was made to Social Services and a section 47 was initiated. This resulted in a case conference being convened. The school nurse liaised with other professionals and then wrote a report identifying her concerns regarding the care of Amy. The particular concerns regarded aspects of neglect which were impacting on both Amy's physical and emotional well-being but the school nurse also recognised that Jon needed help too. A height and weight measurement revealed that Amy had dropped a percentile, and this also caused concerns. The school nurse (SN) spoke to the GP, who was willing to share information with the conference on the family and in particular around Jon's mental health and alcoholism.

The initial case conference

Both Jon and his sister, Hannah, attended the initial case conference and engaged well with the process. Although there was some discussion and disagreement, Amy was subjected to a child protection plan due to neglect. The discussion had centred around the good engagement by Jon and Hannah about the process and that having had these problems bought to public attention they could resolve the problems with help and support. The family recognised that Amy was a child in need.

Management of the case

The extended family was included in the CP plan and Hannah stepped in as a 'role figure' for Amy, visiting often and helping Jon wet comb Amy's hair twice a week. The local church, with which the family had always been connected, became involved and supported Jon in attending alcohol addiction services, with which he engaged very well. Young carers were also involved to support Amy, giving her a regular break. The school nurse worked with Amy in school to build her self-esteem and was also available to Jon, who was grateful for the interventions and talked to the school nurse often. Social care helped Jon to get Amy to school on time. Both Amy and Jon were referred to professional bereavement counsellors to help them deal with Amy's mother's death.

The final outcome for Amy and her family

Amy's father was able to cooperate and engaged in all the services offered. He was relieved to get the help and support that he needed to care for Amy. Amy's general physical appearance improved and she attended school looking well-cared for. The extra support provided by her aunt and the local church, as well as the engagement with young carers meant that she was less anxious, and her schoolwork showed a marked improvement. Specific bereavement work also helped Amy to cope with her mother's death. Amy was removed from the child protection register and became a child in need after six months.

Key issues in this case

- The effects of loss and bereavement on Amy and her father. Often, families can fall apart at the death of a parent.
- The lack of a role model for Amy. Amy was reaching puberty and she needed support from a female adult who she trusted.
- Amy as a young carer. Amy was often responsible not only for her own care but also for that of her father.
- Alcoholism and substance abuse. The impact of this on the lives of children is very significant (Bancroft *et al.*, 2004).
- The success of both statutory and voluntary services working together. In this case good practice achieved satisfactory outcomes for Amy.
- The fact that Amy's father was willing to work with both statutory and voluntary organisations for the benefit of Amy is important.

Early interventions

Bereavement counselling may have been offered to both Amy and her father, and it is important to be aware of the excellent services which work with children and their families following bereavement. These include:

- The Child Bereavement Charity
- Daisy's Dream
- Winston's Wish
- CRUSE

There are still concerns that adult services are reluctant to share information and fail to recognise the significant impact that drug and alcohol misuse can have on a child (Ofsted, 2009). This includes taking on the role of a young carer. It is possible that if more information had been shared, Amy could have been identified as a child in need at a much earlier point and a case conference would not have been required.

Case Study 4.2: Emotional abuse and neglect

Family structure

Ben was five years old at the time of referral and lived with both his parents (Nina and Rafiq), who were not married. Both Nina and Rafiq had been married before and had children who were in their twenties, but not living in the family home. Ben rarely saw his older siblings as they lived a long distance away, and therefore he was effectively an only child. Nina's parents also lived some distance away and they rarely saw Ben or Nina, as there had been a family row after Nina divorced her first husband and moved in with Rafiq. Rafiq's mother was dead, but his father lived close by and was unwell, having had a stroke. Therefore there was little extended family support.

The child protection issue

Nina and Rafiq had a very volatile relationship, often arguing loudly, and neighbours had called the police on many occasions out of concern for Ben's safety. The initial concern was Nina's inability to get Ben to school on time, despite the fact that the family lived within walking distance of the school. Ben was also coming to school hungry, saying he had not had breakfast, and was often unkempt and unwashed. After numerous meetings with the Educational Welfare Officer (EWO) to resolve the situation, a Common Assessment Framework (CAF) referral was sent to Social Services. Nina had real problems around time management and she was invariably late for appointments or did not turn up at all. There were major differences in the parenting style of both parents. Nina found it difficult to set boundaries or have a routine with Ben, but Rafiq was very strict and liked routine. This caused significant conflict between the parents, which in turn impacted on Ben's behaviour. Ben began to present at school with faecal soiling, and he became more withdrawn and tearful at times. He also often looked tired and his concentration levels were very poor, becoming easily distracted and often staring into space. At other times, however, Ben became very angry, hitting other children and staff and often hitting Nina when she came to collect him from school. Nina was unable to manage this aggressive behaviour. She suffered from clinical depression requiring medication. The key issues were around Ben's unpredictable behaviour and soiling in school, in addition to the regular lateness. He was often socially isolated, with few friends, and teachers were struggling to manage him in the classroom.

School nurse involvement
The SN first became involved when Ben started full-time school with a referral from the school in relation to his soiling. After speaking to the GP, a meeting with Ben's parents was arranged and Rafiq attended, but not Nina. It transpired that Ben had suffered from constipation since being a toddler and had been prescribed medication for this on a regular basis. However, Ben often refused to take it and Nina was unable to manage Ben's behaviour well enough to enforce this. The soiling, the unpredictable behaviour and the lateness most mornings were ongoing problems which were impacting on Ben's learning and social development. The school nurse then attempted to undertake some individual parenting work with Nina and Rafiq, but their engagement with the SN was poor and little improvement was made. It was felt, therefore, that a referral needed to be made and an initial case conference was convened. A health assessment was done by the SN for the conference.

The initial case conference
All the reports at the conference were in agreement that the concerns were serious enough for Ben to be subject to a child protection plan as he was suffering from neglect and emotional abuse.

Management of the case
Progress was slow in this case and Ben remained a child in need of protection for two years. This was mainly due to the fact that neither parent engaged with services, and plans to support Ben were often not followed through. Nina's clinical depression meant that she found it increasingly difficult to put Ben's needs first. Over the two years that Ben was on the child protection register, there were a number of changes of social worker, and this was very frustrating. There were concerns about the family's overall mental health and a referral to Child and Adolescent Mental Health Services (CAMHS) was made, but because of poor attendance and non-engagement the family was discharged. The main areas of support from the SN were around Ben's soiling behaviour and managing his anger. The SN liaised with Nina to address the issue of medication, and also with the GP and the paediatrician to establish a care package for Ben, which was successful and significantly improved life for Ben and the family. The school nurse also continued to

work with Ben in school, with Nina and Rafiq's permission, to allow him space and time to talk and establish ways of managing his anger. Agreements with the school and Ben's teachers meant that an anger management strategy could be put in place where Ben could recognise the feelings that he had when he got angry and be able to remove himself from the situation with support from staff.

The final outcome for Ben

Ben was removed from the register after two years. Rafiq moved out of the family home and Ben eventually went to live with him. His school attendance improved once this happened and soiling in school stopped, although he continued to be monitored by the GP. The anger management strategies established by the school nurse and the school in partnership were effective and he began to make friends because he was able to control his anger better, and this helped to improve his overall behaviour. He had contact with Nina infrequently, mainly due to her inability to manage her time as her mental health continued to deteriorate.

Key issues in this case

■ Parental behaviour – in this case it was mainly the behaviour of Nina that seemed to be causing significant problems, although Rafiq's non-engagement was also problematic. Nina had real difficulty in recognising the importance of putting Ben's needs before her own. This may have been related to her personality or her apparently deteriorating mental health. She had no insight into his vulnerability or that her behaviour was having such a detrimental effect on Ben. This may be related to a lack of empathy, her own experience of being parented, poor attachment or a lack of emotional intelligence. These issues can only be addressed if she is helped to recognise the problems and willing to seek appropriate professional treatment and support. The motivation for this can only come from the individual, and unfortunately Nina has not reached this point. There may also have been some family issues that had not been resolved, which were impacting on Nina's mental health. Ben may need support around the 'loss' of his mother as he develops.

■ Soiling – often a result of constipation. It can also be a sign of emotional trauma and also an indicator of sexual abuse (though not in this case). Soiling in school may lead to bullying and a lack of friendships, which impacts on social and emotional development. Teachers may also be angry about having to sort out this problem. It is important for the SN to be an advocate for the child and ensure that the school staff understand the issues and that good care packages are in place with roles clearly defined.

■ Behavioural issues – Ben began his school career being late into the classroom most days. This impacts on social development because there are limited opportunities to make friends. It also means he stands out as different from the others. Neglect was also impacting on his behaviour and his tiredness may have been due to a poor diet or maybe a lack of sleep due to poor bedtime routines.

■ Chaotic parenting techniques – a lack of boundaries and routine cause anxiety in children. In particular, both parents using different styles of parenting is confusing for a child and impacts on their social and emotional development.

Early intervention
Earlier interventions in this case would rely on the identification of problems sooner. Nina's mental health problems might have been identified earlier. It is possible that she had suffered from post-natal depression, which was not resolved, and this may have led to poor attachment.

Access to advice and support on parenting for both parents would have been very beneficial, but this was a family who found it difficult to engage with services.

Again, it is important for all agencies to be sharing information when a child is at risk of harm. The school intervened early by notifying the educational welfare services and the school nurse of their concerns, and this is important for early identification of need. The HCP recommends good communication between health visitors and school health teams and any information about the family should be passed on to the school nurse.

Case study 4.3: Physical abuse and domestic violence

Family structure
Tom was 14 and Stephen 13 at the time of referral. Tom's father, Mike, died when Tom was 1, and Tom's mother, Sally, had suffered from depression since then; she was on medication for this. Sally had a supportive network of extended family who had been very good when Mike died, and Tom had apparently coped very well with his father's death.

When Tom was 14, Sally met Dan on the Internet while he was in prison for assaulting his first wife. Dan had two children, Stephen 13, and Jodie

9. Dan had separated from his first wife and Stephen had chosen to live with Dan. Stephen saw his mum and Jodie occasionally, but they had moved some distance away to be closer to family. Stephen had wanted to stay at his school with his friends and to be near his grandparents. There was a clear history of domestic violence fuelled by alcohol with Dan's first wife. While Dan was in prison, Stephen lived with his paternal grandparents who lived nearby and to whom he had a strong attachment.

Dan and Sally married five months after meeting and Dan and Stephen moved into Sally's small council flat; Tom and Stephen shared a bedroom.

The child protection issue

The relationship between Sally and Dan quickly became volatile and there were soon reports of domestic violence made by neighbours and also by Sally. These were received by the safeguarding team and disseminated to the most appropriate members of staff. These reports were mostly linked to physical violence by Dan towards Sally, often associated with heavy drinking. However, some reports were also about Dan self-harming by cutting his arms in front of the children. Sally was then leaving the boys to take Dan to the hospital for treatment. Children's Social Care carried out a section 47 enquiry and an initial case conference was called.

School nurse involvement

Both boys were seen prior to conference for a health assessment, including height, weight, vision and hearing by the SN, all of which were satisfactory. A holistic assessment was carried out, exploring their thoughts and feelings about the family situation. They both disclosed that they had witnessed family arguments, and that Dan drank heavily and sometimes cut himself. They also expressed concerns about Sally's safety and that she was often crying and sad. Stephen had clearly formed a good relationship with Sally. Tom said he resented Dan in the family home, but he liked Stephen and they got on well together. He also said he felt safe because he thought that Sally would always protect him.

The initial case conference

The level of domestic violence in this case was sufficiently high that it was a unanimous decision that both boys should be subjects of a protection plan. The school nurse noted that the risk to the boys was high for emotional abuse, as they were both witnessing the arguments between Dan and Sally. The boys had expressed concern over Sally, wanting to protect her, and this put them at risk of physical harm as well. Stephen was now calling her 'Mum' and had formed a strong attachment to her. Although neither boy at this time had been physically abused, there were considerable concerns raised that they may be caught in the 'cross fire' especially as they had both expressed the wish to protect Sally.

The plan consisted of:

- Regular visits by the social worker
- Sally to attend a group for victims of domestic abuse
- Dan to attend a perpetrators' group; however, he would not admit he was a perpetrator
- Dan to attend local drug action team to help with his alcohol use
- Both parents to have parenting support
- The children were referred for an assessment by CAMHS

Management of the case

Initially the plan progressed well. Sally engaged with the process from the outset and Dan could see the benefit that his cooperation might help them to gain a bigger property through the local authority housing department. Dan did not acknowledge any problems with violence towards women. There was another violent incident where Stephen was hurt while trying to protect Sally. Sally was praised for then removing both herself and the boys from the flat to safety. Stephen made a statement to the police and it was agreed that he would return to his grandparents' home. From Stephen's perspective he had not done anything wrong and was now being penalised for his behaviour and this has had a hugely detrimental effect on his emotional wellbeing. Sally later retracted her statement and Stephen then wanted to retract his statement as well. However, the police still prosecuted Dan. He was given a two-year suspended sentence and Stephen continued to live with his paternal grandparents.

Sally then became pregnant. The next case conference was brought forward to include a pre-conference for the unborn baby. Studies show that a pregnant woman is at increased risk of significant harm where the partner has a history of domestic violence. Children's social care also started to explore the legal aspects of removing Tom and Stephen and the baby at birth and requested a full parenting and psychological report to be undertaken. This report was conducted over several days and identified that Sally and Dan were codependent. This meant that Sally needs to 'mother' and take care of Dan just as much as he is 'controlling' in his behaviour towards her. However, there was not enough evidence to remove the children or the newborn baby. Dan reduced his alcohol intake, but became addicted to prescription drugs taken for a bad back.

The risks remain very high, especially to Sally and Cameron, the new baby. However, there have not now been any reported incidents for many months and even though the psychological report is quite damning there may not be sufficient evidence to remove any of the children. It is felt that Tom and Stephen have enough resilience now that any attempts to transfer them into foster care may be more harmful than leaving them where they are. There remain concerns that the dynamics within the family are still such that an incident in the future may well end in tragedy. Sally lost her extended family, as they do not like Dan, and she may end up feeling very isolated. Another complicating factor is her own mental health, which means that she is also taking medication. She does have a good insight into her relationship and the hope is that she can continue to utilise available services to help her manage the relationship. Stephen now has permission to spend some nights with his dad and Sally, but does not access this as much as he is allowed. Both boys adore their baby brother (Cameron) and are very good with him.

The final outcome for the children

After some problems early on in the plan, the family eventually undertook all of the actions required of them to fulfil the elements of the child protection plan. There have not been any reported incidents for a significant length of time. There are not sufficient reasons to continue a plan; however, the risks remain high. This creates a huge dilemma for the school nurse, who needs to continue to support Stephen and Tom in the school setting and be vigilant of escalating concerns. There is a drop-in at the school and both Stephen and Tom call in from time to time, having built a relationship with the SN. The SN also works closely with the health visitor with responsibility for Sally and Cameron to monitor the situation there.

Key issues to consider

- Mental health problems with both Dan and Sally and the use of substances: prescription drugs and alcohol.
- Loss and bereavement issues for everyone, either through the death of Mike or the separation of Dan and his first wife.
- Family relationships and the dynamics of 'blended' families.
- Domestic violence and the impact on young people's development and the increased risks associated with pregnancy.
- The psychological aspects of codependency: why abused individuals stay with abusers.
- The difficulties of older children on child protection plans and how this is managed.

- Adolescent development and the transition into adulthood and being a parent.

Early intervention
- Early intervention with Sally's possible post-natal depression and professional bereavement counselling may have raised her resilience and reduced her vulnerability.
- Multi-agency working with regard to Dan's problems; rehabilitation through the prison services and help with his drinking problems. The problem is that individuals need to be ready to change their behaviour and perhaps having baby Cameron was the motivation to change for Dan.
- It is important to be aware of the number of young people who are in violent relationships and consider this to be acceptable (Barter *et al.*, 2009). There is a role for school nurses to be actively involved in sex and relationship education throughout the school year to promote healthy, loving relationships (see Chapter 5).

Case study 4.4: Sexual abuse

Family structure and background
Jenny was 15 at the time of the referral. She attended the local secondary school, where the school nurse ran a drop-in. Jenny lived at home with her mother (Jane) and two younger siblings: Freya, aged 10, and Kevin, aged 13. Kevin also attended the same school as Jenny. When Jenny was 14, her parents separated and her father left the country to live in Australia with his new partner, so Jenny rarely sees him. Jenny attended the drop-in at the time of the divorce for support from the school nurse and school counsellor, as she was struggling to deal with her father not only leaving home but also moving so far away. She had found the support at the drop-in very helpful. Jenny's mother (Jane) started a new relationship with Greg six months after the divorce from Jenny's father, which Jenny found very difficult to cope with. Greg then moved into the family home about three months after the relationship began. Having established a good relationship with the school nurse, Jenny continued to have regular contact and attended the drop-in regularly for support. Jenny began to come more frequently to the drop-in and displayed signs of anxiety, which gradually increased.

The child protection issue

At one of the drop-in sessions, Jenny disclosed that when they are alone, Greg made inappropriate comments to her and that he had tried to fondle her breasts. She was clearly very upset but did not want to tell her mother, as they had been rowing frequently and Jane had called her a troublemaker who resented her being happy with Greg. Jane had also just started working at the local supermarket in the evenings, leaving the children with Greg. Jenny was worried that both Kevin and Freya would be vulnerable if she went out and left them alone with Greg.

School nurse involvement

The school nurse explained that she would have to share this information. She made a referral to the Children and Families' team in Social Care and also spoke to her named nurse for child protection. Jane was informed, and after Greg was told to leave the house she came to the school to collect Jenny. As soon as Jenny had left the room the SN made clear and detailed notes of what had been said. Following a section 47 enquiry a case conference was convened. The SN did an appropriate health assessment on all three children and submitted her report. She shared the report with Jane and appropriate parts with Jenny.

The initial case conference

Jane and Jenny both attended the case conference. Jane had been very shocked by the disclosure, but immediately supportive of Jenny and concerned for the welfare of Kevin and Freya. She was angry with Greg, but also felt very guilty that she had put them in danger by allowing a man she did not know very well to come and live in her house. Greg was continuing to be investigated by the police and there had been previous allegations of sexual offences, but not with underage women. As Jane had agreed not to have any further contact with Greg and an injunction had been taken out to prevent him coming within close proximity of the family home, it was deemed that the children were at no risk of harm at the present time.

The conference did make recommendations that the family should receive support from CAMHS.

Jenny was encouraged to continue to use the drop-in at the school for support when she felt the need.

The final outcome for the children

All three children were assessed by CAMHS, but it was felt that only Jenny required ongoing therapy. She engaged well and she was able to refocus on her school work, achieving well in her exams. Jane did become depressed, but after counselling and support from her GP she now has a daytime job.

Early intervention

The fact that Jenny was able to disclose to the school nurse at an early stage could be seen as one reason that there was such a positive outcome. She had already built up a trusting relationship and was aware of an appropriate, trusted adult to talk to. The school nurse listened and responded appropriately, minimising the harm to all the children.

Key issues in this case

Young people need to be listened to and be believed about what is happening to them. In this case both the SN and Jane believed Jenny. This is not always the case, and relationships such as Jane and Greg's can survive through extreme circumstances (see previous case).

Jenny is 15, and often this age of adolescence can be extremely difficult in terms of social care. At this age of transition into adulthood, if removal from the home is necessary, placements with foster carers can be problematic. Young people in difficult circumstances may run away, become homeless, form inappropriate relationships or become involved in prostitution or illicit substances.

School nurses have the potential to support these young people and act as advocate for them. They can also help to build resilience and self-esteem, which are crucial to the emotional development of adolescents.

Conclusion

The case studies provide a few examples of the complex family situations which may lead to children being at risk of significant harm. Within their work, school nurses will need to respond to a variety of situations: sometimes immediately, and at other times after consultation with their colleagues. It is important to consider the myriad of risks to young people's safety in different environments as they grow in independence. It is also important to have an understanding of child development so that school nurses are able to make sensible assessments of risk.

With the widening use of social networking, children are becoming increasingly vulnerable. They need to be aware of the dangers they may be exposing themselves to. This was emphasised in the review carried out by Byron (2008), and her recommendations included the importance of educating children about the dangers they can encounter. The school nurse should see this as a part of their public health role within the communities in which they work (see Chapter 3).

Practitioners also need to be aware of other groups of children who may be living in the community in which they are working. Firstly, there are those who are not attending school. This may be because of legitimately approved home schooling, but there are also those who continually fail to attend or who have been excluded.

It is also important to be aware of the growing problem of child trafficking, which the NSPCC (2011) defines as 'the recruitment and movement of children for the purpose of exploitation'. These children will be used for commercial gain, often in the sex industry or in the drug trade. It is important to follow up any concerns, especially when there are inconsistencies in addresses or deliberate vagueness by children or their carers of the next of kin (HM Government, 2008b).

It is estimated that around 20,000 girls under the age of 15 are at risk of female genital mutilation each year (HM Government, 2011). The age that this procedure is often carried out is between five and eight (London Safeguarding Board, 2009). It is important to consider those children who are most likely to be at risk and be aware of national and local guidelines. The *Multi-Agency Practice Guidelines: Female Genital Mutilation* (HM Government, 2011) are very comprehensive and should be read and kept available for reference by all health workers working with women and children in the community.

In summary, the key aspects of effective child protection practice are:

- Awareness of the current national and local guidelines and procedures.
- Attendance at regular Interagency child protection training.
- Clear, accurate, contemporaneous and comprehensive record-keeping.
- Discuss any concerns with the named nurse for child protection in your area.
- When making referrals, be clear about your concerns and use evidence from your knowledge of child development theory and research on the impact of abuse to inform your recommendations within your reports for child protection.
- Be clear about your role and what is appropriate for you to be responsible for in the child protection plan.
- Share information appropriately and work in partnership.
- Use child protection supervision both to improve practice and provide yourself with essential emotional support.
- And most importantly, listen to the child and young person and ensure their needs are the focus of any discussions. Be an advocate for the child.

References

Bancroft, A., Wilson, S., Cunningham-Burley, S., Becket-Milburn, K. and Masters, H. (2004) *Parental Drug and Alcohol Misuse. Resilience and Transition Among Young People.* Joseph Rowntree Foundation, York.

Barlow, J. and Calam, R. (2011) A public health approach to safeguarding in the 21st century. *Child Abuse Review*, **20**, 238–55.

Barter, G., Mc Carry, M., Berridge, D. and Evans, K. (2009) *Partner Exploitation and Violence in Teenage Intimate Relationships.* NSPCC, London.

Byron, T. (2008) *Safer Children in a Digital World.* DCFS, London.

Daniel, B., Taylor, J., Scott, J., Derbyshire, D. and Neilson, D. (2011) *Recognising and Helping the Neglected Child.* Jessica Kingsley, London.

Department for Education (2010) *Working Together to Safeguard Children. A Guide to to Inter-agency Working to Safeguard and Promote the Welfare of Children.* DE, London.

Department of Health (2012) *Getting it Right for Children, Young People and Their Families. Maximising the Contribution of the School Nursing Team. Vision and Call to Action.* DH, London.

Department of Health/Department for Children, Schools and Families (2009) *The Healthy Child Programme from 5 to 19.* DH/DCSF, London.

Ford, S. (2009) School nurses increasingly taking on child protection work. *Nursing Times*, 19 May. Available at http://www.nursingtimes.net/whats-new-in-nursing/rcn-congress/school-nurses-increasingly-taking-on-child-protection-work/5001599.article (accessed 4 January 2012).

HM Government (2008a) *Information Sharing: Guidance for Practitioners and Managers.* The Stationery Office, London.

HM Government (2008b) *Safeguarding Children Who May Have Been Trafficked.* The Stationery Office, London.

HM Government (2011) *Multi-Agency Practice Guidelines: Female Genital Mutilation.* The Stationery Office, London.

Laming, L. (2009) *The Protection of Children in England: A Progress Report.* The Stationery Office, London.

London Safeguarding Board (2009) *London Female Genital Mutilation Resource Pack.* London Safeguarding Board, London.

Munro, E. (2008) *Effective Child Protection*, 2nd edn. Sage, London.

Munro, E. (2011) *The Munro Review of Child Protection. Final Report. A Child-centred System.* Department of Education, London.

National Society for the Prevention of Cruelty to Children [NSPCC] (2011) *Child Trafficking.* Available at http://www.nspcc.org.uk/ (accessed 19 March 2012).

Nursing and Midwifery Council (2008) *The Code. Standards of Conduct, Performance and*

Ethics for Nurses and Midwives. NMC, London.

Office for Standards in Education, Children's Services and Skills (2009) *Learning Lessons From Serious Case Reviews*. Ofsted, London.

Office for Standards in Education, Children's Services and Skills (2011) *The Voice of the Child: Learning Lessons From Serious Case Reviews. Year 2*. Ofsted, London.

Royal College of Paediatrics and Child Health (2010) *Safeguarding Children and Young People: Roles and Competences for Health Care Staff. Intercollegiate Document*. RCP-CH, London.

Stafford, A., Vincent, S. and Parton,N. (2010) *Child Protection Reform Across the UK*. Dunedin, Edinburgh.

Trodd, L. and Chivers, L. (2011) *Interprofessional Working in Practice. Learning and Working Together for Children and Families*. Open University Press, Maidenhead.

CHAPTER 5

Contributing to Personal, Social, Health and Economic education (PSHE)

Melanie Hayward

Key themes in this chapter:

- What is the policy behind health education in child centred public health?
- What is the PSHE Education Curriculum?
- Why should School nurses be involved with PSHE Education?
- What should be taught at which stage of the curriculum?
- How do you assess need in relation to PSHE?
- Who else can contribute to PSHE programmes from the school health team?
- Valuing difference and diversity
- Planning PSHE education
- Delivering PSHE education
- Sex and Relationships Education (SRE)

Introduction

Personal, Social, Health and Economic education (PSHE education) is a developmental programme of learning intended to help children and young people acquire the knowledge, understanding and skills they need to manage their lives, now and in the future. Between the ages of 5 and 19 years, children and young people experience inherent emotional and physical changes which are influenced by many internal and external factors. Debell and Jackson (2000) describe this as a 'metamorphosis', from dependence to independence. The perceived benefits of PSHE education are widespread and it should aim to support all children and young people, whatever their individual circumstances. The aim of this chapter is to examine the school nurse's role in PSHE education. Arguably, PSHE education has the potential to make a major contribution to children and young people's health and wellbeing, helping them achieve independence and a positive future (PSHE Association, 2011). In the UK, there are significant health issues reported which affect young people, such as childhood obesity, teenage pregnancy and 'binge' drinking (Adamson, 2007). School nurses are ideally placed to contribute to PSHE programmes because they are a link between health, education and social services. PSHE education has the potential to contribute to the long-term health of the nation, which in turn helps to reduce National Health Service (NHS) spending (Hayward, 2011).

What is the policy behind health education in child-centred public health?

It is argued that many of the health issues facing young people today are a result of lifestyle choices. Behaviours including poor diet, lack of exercise, smoking, drinking alcohol, drug misuse and other risk-taking behaviours contribute to conditions such as eating disorders, sexually transmitted infections and mental health problems. Experience suggests that just telling a population how to be healthy is not enough to initiate behaviour change, but ensuring that young people get the information they need to make sensible decisions about their future lives and supporting them through those choices has the potential to be very effective.

A number of policy documents in recent years have focused on the health and social needs of children and young people:

- The *Every Child Matters Programme* (DH/DfES, 2004) set out an approach to achieve health and wellbeing for all children, with health education playing a major role in these outcomes.
- *Choosing Health* (DH, 2004a) and *Our Health, Our Care, Our Say* (DH, 2006) provided further policy direction for public health improvement, given impetus through the Wanless Report (Wanless, 2004), advocating a fully engaged approach to sustained health improvement.
- *The Children's Plan* (DCSF, 2007) pledged to improve educational attainment through promoting and developing personal and social skills and reducing risky behaviour, which can lead to poor health.
- The *Youth Alcohol Action Plan* (DH/DCSF, 2008a) was launched from *The Children's Plan* and aimed to reduce the occurrence of teenage drinking by providing clear information to parents about the risks and encouraging education in schools to enable young people to make better decisions regarding alcohol use. This was complemented by the 'Why let drink decide?' national media campaign, providing all levels of practical advice such as how to be in control of drinking and guidance on looking after a drunken friend.

- The *Healthy Weight, Healthy Lives* (DH/DCSF, 2008b) strategy was aimed at persuading parents to improve their children's diet and increase their physical activity through campaigns such as *Change4Life*. It also encouraged health education in school, with messages such as the 'five a day' fruit and vegetable campaign and a reintroduction of cooking lessons and walking buses linked to the *PE and Sports Strategy for Young People* (DCSF, 2008). The aim of this strategy was to increase the amount of physical activity in schools.
- The *Teenage Pregnancy Strategy* (Social Exclusion Unit [SEU], 1999) set out to tackle both the causes and consequences of teenage pregnancy, with health education playing a major part in both targeted interventions and general teaching in schools. Media campaigns such as *RUThinking?* (DfES, 2007) and *Want Respect? Use a Condom* were used to raise awareness in young people. In 2001, the Government published the *National Strategy for Sexual Health and HIV* (DH, 2001) setting out an ambitious 10-year programme to tackle sexual ill health. In terms of health education this involved providing clear information so that young people could make informed decisions about preventing STIs, different types of contraception, safe sex and how they can access local sources of further advice and treatment.
- The *Healthy Lives, Brighter Futures* (DH/DSCF, 2009a) child strategy built on the National Service Frameworks (DH, 2004b) and professionals were encouraged to provide support and information to enable children and young people to lead healthier lives through motivation and empowerment.
- The *Healthy Child Programme* (DH/DCSF, 2009b) is the programme outlining recommendations for this universal service at local practice level and recommends the different roles and responsibilities of health practitioners within it.

Schools are increasingly recognised as the ideal place for promoting the health and social skills of children and young people. Both *Healthy Lives, Healthy People* (HM Government, 2010) and *The Importance of Teaching* (DE, 2010) continued to endorse health and pastoral care within schools and identify PSHE education as a central theme. School nurses continue to provide expertise and local health knowledge in order to meet identified health priorities and help schools develop as 'health-promoting environments' (HM Government, 2010, p. 36).

What is the PSHE education curriculum?

The school curriculum comprises all learning and other experiences that each school plans for its pupils. PSHE education has been part of the National Curriculum within the UK for over 10 years and is intended to support pupils' learning and personal development. The subject areas taught within PSHE education and related policy differ across England, Scotland, Wales and Northern Ireland; this chapter relates to the English context. PSHE education is not a statutory subject and schools do not have to provide it. However, schools are required to contribute to the personal and social development of their pupils through the promotion of moral, mental and physical development in order to prepare them for the responsibilities and experiences of adult life (DfES, 2004). Schools are required to have policies that relate to many of the aspects of personal development, such as sex and relationship education, bullying, drugs in school and safeguarding. These policies are overarching statutory requirements for all state-maintained schools and the knowledge and skills relating to the behaviours required to realise these are developed through frameworks of PSHE. The laws in 2012 remain confusing: the clauses that would have made PSHE statutory within the Children's, Schools and Families Bill were removed as a result of the negotiations in April 2011, so schools still do not have to provide it (Hayward, 2011). There are statutory topics in the curriculum, such as sexual health, drugs and alcohol or work-related advice, that are covered in other subject areas, but there is no requirement to have a separate PSHE framework, although many schools do (QCA, 1999). There are also differences between the current legal status of Sex and Relationships Education (SRE) within academy, free and state maintained schools. Even though the establishment of academies and free schools differs and they are funded in the same way, they are not required to have an up-to-date SRE policy or teach SRE (Sex Education Forum [SEF], 2011a).

The Qualifications Curriculum Authority's (QCA) review of the secondary curriculum (QCA, 2007) asked schools to look creatively at timetabling for all areas of the curriculum. There are great pressures on the curriculum, so schools need to allocate curriculum time on the basis of pupil need. Many schools are beginning to bring subjects together to offer a more creative approach to learning. What is important is that pupils have regular access to high-quality PSHE experiences. In January 2011 the government announced a major review into the National Curriculum (DE, 2011) which excluded PSHE. There followed an internal review to evaluate how schools could be supported to improve the quality of PSHE teaching. This included ongoing flexibility for teachers to use their judgment about how best to deliver PSHE education across all key stages. The Government's decision for a separate internal review was in recognition that good PSHE education supports individual children and young people to make safe and informed choices and that schools often need external help with the more sensitive topics (DE, 2010). It could be argued that if PSHE education was given statutory status, starting in primary education, there would be earlier opportunities for preventative work.

In 2010 an Ofsted report showed that most pupils enjoyed their PSHE lessons and saw their relevance (Ofsted, 2010). The development of personal and social skills was a particular strength. Young people generally knew how to stay safe and healthy, although not all of them applied this knowledge to the decisions they made. This is where school nurses can make a difference, as they have understanding of the real issues and concerns that children and young people face and can provide appropriate ongoing support if necessary (Emmerson, 2011).

Why should school nurses be involved with PSHE education?

The Healthy Schools Programme was designed to promote a holistic approach to health within education through core themes of PSHE education. The Healthy School agenda bridges the gap between the health and educational workforces, and school nurses are recognised within the literature as having a lead role (Health Development Agency, 2002). Ofsted (2007) recognised that schools with the most effective PSHE curriculum have developed constructive links with other support services, such as school nursing, that can provide not only health education but ongoing advice and support. The role of the school nurse complements that of teachers because school nurses act as health advisors to children, parents, teachers and others and they have information on other local health services (Hayward, 2011).

Research and policy indicate that the benefits of school nurse involvement in PSHE education are:

- **School nurses have unique insight into the health needs of school communities**. Caan (2010) and Kennedy (2010) state that school nurses pursue positive health outcomes for children and young people by appreciating the wider context of public health. Marmot (2010, p. 24) emphasised the need for a '...collaborative school based workforce, working across school-home boundaries if real and sustainable success is to be achieved through health education'.
- **School nurses have expert and up-to-date knowledge of health issues**. Whilst teachers have the skills for teaching, they do not always have the required expert knowledge or confidence to deliver specialised or sensitive topics. Some of the public health issues that young people face are concerning and often seem overwhelming to deal with for teachers who may not have health promotion knowledge and skills (Hayward, 2011). Research undertaken by the NSPCC (2009) indicated that young people felt that teachers did not

take health education seriously and that they did not have the expert knowledge to discuss the issues that could be raised. School nurses are highly-skilled and qualified in helping children and young people choose and maintain healthy lifestyles.

- **School nurses are comfortable discussing sensitive topics such as body parts and sexual activity**. Practice indicates that there may be a reluctance from teachers to teach some topics, for example, sex and relationships education (SRE). Teachers may not feel that it is appropriate for them to teach SRE to their pupils for a number of reasons. When a teacher shows embarrassment this is quickly recognised by pupils and they can become embarrassed themselves or react negatively to the subject. School nurses are accustomed to discussing sensitive topics and can therefore confidently present these types of subjects (Hayward, 2011). Schools may also acknowledge that young people will feel more comfortable asking questions of a health professional rather than someone who teaches them other subjects within the school setting.

- **School nurses have a non-judgmental and informal teaching style conducive to discussing sensitive topics**. Young people have stated that much of the content of teacher-led health education lessons is not very interesting, is not communicated at their level and does not engage them in the issues that matter to them (NSPCC, 2009). According to Ofsted (2010), inadequate lessons are mainly taught by form tutors, who may lack the necessary expertise to engage pupils and to challenge their misconceptions. External agencies are highlighted as valuable in providing expert contributions which can enliven lessons (Ofsted, 2010).

- **School nurses allow discussion of controversial matters as well as personal consultation for pupils who do not wish to share with school or parents**. School nurses work under the NMC Code (NMC, 2008) and use Fraser guidelines to guide their practice, which is different from how teachers work (see Chapter 6). If personal issues arise within a PSHE session, school nurses have the expertise to address these on a one-to-one basis and do not have the constraints of the timings of a school day (Hayward, 2011).

- **School nurses can provide PSHE education in a variety of settings and groups, as well as one-to-one consultation**. School nurses can cross the barriers between school, home and other settings. This means that as well as requested curricula-based sessions at school they can provide sessions to meet identified needs within school or other venues such as youth groups; they can also work with specific client sets such as single sex or vulnerable groups. Research shows that SRE can have more impact if taught in small groups (Emmerson, 2011), but teachers often do not have the capacity for this. School nurses are not constrained by lesson times, so are able to provide a more tailored service on a one-to-one or small group basis if necessary (see Chapter 2). School nurses can also provide support for parents and carers to enable them to be health educators for their children (Hayward, 2011).

What should be taught at which stage of the curriculum?

The National Curriculum is organised on the basis of four key stages. The Education Act (HMSO, 1996, section 353b) sets out what pupils should be taught at each key stage and attainment targets are set. It is for schools to choose how they organise their school curriculum to include the programmes of study and plan their schemes of work.

Key Stage 1: ages 5 to 7 years

- Pupils learn about themselves as developing individuals and as members of their communities, building on their own experiences and on the early learning goals for personal, social and emotional development.
- They learn the basic rules and skills for keeping themselves healthy and safe and for behaving well. They have opportunities to show they can take some responsibility for themselves and their environment.
- They begin to learn about their own and other people's feelings and become aware of the views, needs and rights of other children and older people.
- As members of a class and school community, they learn social skills such as how to share, take turns, play, help others, resolve simple arguments and resist bullying. They begin to take an active part in the life of their school and the community.

Specific areas where school nurses can contribute to the curriculum are:

- How to make simple choices to improve their health and wellbeing, e.g. healthy diet and exercise.
- How and why to maintain personal hygiene.
- How diseases are spread and can be controlled.
- Processes of growing from young to old and how a person's needs change.
- Naming parts of the body.
- Understanding that all household products, including medicines, can be harmful if not used properly.
- Rules for keeping safe and how people can help them stay safe.
- Identifying safe adults to talk to.

Key Stage 2: ages 7 to 11 years

- Pupils learn about themselves as growing and changing individuals with their own experiences and ideas and as members of their communities.
- They develop their sense of social justice and moral responsibility and begin to understand that their own choices and behaviour can affect local, national or global issues and political and social institutions.
- As they begin to develop into young adults, they face the changes of puberty and transfer to secondary school with support and encouragement from their school.
- They learn how to make more confident and informed choices about their health and environment; to take more responsibility, individually and as a group, for their own learning; and to resist bullying.

Specific areas where school nurses can contribute to the curriculum are:

- What a healthy lifestyle is, both physical and emotional.
- Understanding how bacteria and viruses affect health and how safe routines reduce their spread.
- How the body changes during puberty, how emotions change at that time and how to deal with their feelings towards themselves, their family and others in a positive way.
- Legal and illegal substances and their effects.
- How to recognise different risks and how to behave responsibly, judging what kind of physical contact is acceptable or unacceptable.
- How to resist pressure to do wrong and how to ask for help.
- Basic first aid.

Key Stages 3 and 4: ages 11 to 16 years

At this stage, PSHE education includes work-related topics such as careers, enterprise and financial capability. For the purpose of this chapter the focus is on personal wellbeing.

- Pupils learn about healthy lifestyles and the wellbeing of others.
- They develop an understanding that physical and emotional health affects the ability to lead fulfilling lives and that there is help and support available.
- They learn that dealing with growth and change are normal parts of growing up.
Specific areas where school nurses can contribute to the curriculum are:
- Key Stage 3: ages 11 to 14 years
  - Physical and emotional aspects of puberty.

- Sexual activity, reproduction, contraception, pregnancy, sexually transmitted infections and HIV.
- How high-risk behaviours affect health and wellbeing.
- Facts about drug, alcohol and tobacco use and the personal and social consequences.
- How making choices for healthy living contributes to personal wellbeing.
- Develop social skills of communication, negotiation and assertiveness.

■ Key Stage 4: ages 14 to 16 years
- How the media portray young people, body image and health issues.
- The characteristics of emotional and mental health, causes, symptoms and treatments of some mental health problems.
- Benefits and risks of lifestyle choices, including sexual activity and substance misuse and the short- and long-term health consequences.
- Where and how to obtain health information and ways to reduce risk and minimise harm.
- Basic first and emergency aid.
- Characteristics of positive relationships, and awareness of exploitation in relationships and of organisations that support relationships in crisis.
- Parenting skills and qualities and their central importance to family life.
- Impact of separation, divorce and bereavement on families and the need to adapt to changing circumstances.

How do you assess need in relation to PSHE?

The principles of assessing need are discussed in other chapters. However, in relation to PSHE, it is important to have an awareness of the general needs of the specific school population as well as the broader community in order to provide relevant topics within the PSHE programmes. Needs assessment can also be described as school health profiling or planning and involves the collection of health, social and economic data locally and nationally (see Chapter 7) (Gleeson, 2001). This evidence is then used to develop school health action plans which will provide information on what the school health team will do in the school community to improve health. This will include all health promotion, prevention and surveillance activities as well as PSHE. School nurses will need to develop a template or tool to help collect the data. NICE identifies a step-by-step approach for health needs assessment (NICE, 2005). The RCN toolkit (RCN, 2008) also sets out ideas of what should be included and how this can be best presented to ensure user friendliness.

PSHE education needs can be highlighted in a number of ways:

- A specific issue raised by the school, for example, a PSHE session may be undertaken within a form group, where a pupil has been diagnosed with a specific condition.
- An increase in teenage pregnancy in the school.
- A rise in the number of pupils accessing A&E for emergency contraception.
- A rise in reported bullying.
- An increase in the numbers accessing a drop-in at the school.
- Raised levels of truancy.
- Discovery of alcohol, smoking or drugs in the school.
- High levels of obesity highlighted by the child weight measurement programme.
- Requests from pupils or teachers.
- Local health data will include the particular public health concerns of the community, such as high levels of dental caries (see Table 5.1).

Who else can contribute to PSHE programmes from the school health team?

School nurses lead the school health teams across the country, and models will vary as we have seen in previous chapters. However, it is evident that PSHE is not necessarily delivered by qualified SCPHNs but by members of a mixed skill team including community staff nurses (CSNs), nursery nurses (NNs) and school health assistants (SHAs). A negative view is often proffered about skill mix, with claims of a 'diluted service' and qualified SCPHNs being fearful of losing their professional identity. In fact, literature shows a mixed picture of skill mix, with a lack of valid and reliable research from the community public health setting (SNMAC, 2002). In many areas, skill mix is very effectively utilised to enable school nurses to focus on the needs of the community. PSHE education is a role that, given training in presentation and facilitation skills and encouragement, most members of the school nursing team can undertake. Specific training using the PSHE Continuing Professional Development (CPD) course would also be beneficial not just for CSNs and NNs but school nurses as well.

Re-drawing boundaries between job roles is a complicated organisational challenge and research shows that much depends on the ability of the leader to manage the change, alongside staff attitude (Hyde *et al.*, 2005). The impact of workforce modernisation on staff remains controversial, and resistance to change is a common phenomenon (Tomey, 2004). These issues are discussed further in Chapter 3.

Table 5.1 Assessing need (sources: NICE, 2005, p. 12; Blair *et al.*, 2003; Stevens and Gilliam, 1998).

Skills	Methods	Example using oral health
Epidemiological assessment		
■ Compare demography and health status of the target population	Examination of local demographic knowledge from various sources, for example: *Public health observatories National statistics Health Survey for England Neighbourhood statistics Local authority Healthy Schools Teams Safeguarding teams Local NHS services School*	Collect information on oral health using: *National statistics Health Survey for England Public health observatories Children's Dental Health in the United Kingdom Reports Local safeguarding teams – children with oral health problems Local dental services/dentists Local A&E and hospital attendance for dental caries School – absent figures related to dental issues Health questionnaires/screening*
Comparative assessment		
■ Contrast services available locally with those available to similar populations in other areas ■ Contrast services by other providers	Examination of other services that provide health promotion within the school, local area and other areas. Asking questions such as: *Does this need get serviced by other agencies? If so how appropriate and effective is it? Could school nursing provide more appropriate PSHE? Or fill any gaps where it isn't being taught? Should school nursing be providing PSHE alongside other professionals?*	Collect information asking questions such as: *Do local oral/dental services provide PSHE resources or sessions within schools? Within this school? With which pupils? How often? What's the content of the sessions? How are they evaluated by schools/ pupils?*
Corporate assessment		
■ Gathers views, desires, and knowledge of others	Examine national and regional and local priorities: *Department of Health Department of Education National Curriculum Ofsted NICE* Examine local commissioning/ management service targets: *Local authority Local NHS services Children's Trust* Consider others with special knowledge other agencies, children, young people and parents	National Priorities such as: *Valuing People's Oral Health* (DH, 2007a), *Smokefree and Smiling* (DH, 2007b), *Choosing Better Oral Health: Oral Health Plan for England* (DH, 2005), *Delivering Better Oral Health: an Evidence-based Toolkit for Prevention* (DH/BASCD, 2009) Local priorities such as: *Public health reports, Healthy Child Programme, School Nursing Service priorities* Others, for example: *Information gathered through a variety of qualitative methods such as; focus groups or questionnaires.*

How does PSHE education fit in with traditional health promotion models?

There are a number of health promotion approaches and models and PSHE best fits in the 'education approach', which aims to provide individuals with knowledge, understanding and skills so that they can make informed decisions. Health education can be described as being limited in that it may provide knowledge without the 'enabling' elements of health promotion (Nutbeam, 2000). School nurses may be providing 'one-off' sessions with one opportunity to provide information, and it may be necessary to ensure that at least one key message is established. Ideally, school nurses will be involved on a spiral curriculum with more opportunities to build relationships and empower children and young people to make the right choices regarding their health. PSHE education should help pupils to explore their feelings, build confidence, promote self-esteem and encourage self-determination, and school nurses may only have one opportunity to inspire young people to seek more help if necessary (Naidoo and Wills, 2005). Table 5.2 shows how the education approach can be used in sexual health.

An 'asset model' can be applied to PSHE where health is seen as an achievable and valuable asset and positive abilities are promoted, rather than focusing on the negative aspects of 'diseases' (Morgan and Ziglio, 2007). So, for example,

Table 5.2 An example of using the educational approach in PSHE education focusing on sexual health.

Delivery methods	Activities	Nurse/client relationship	Intended outcomes
Presentation of information	PowerPoint, DVDs/ videos, computer programmes, talk	School nurse-led	To increase knowledge
Exploration of attitudes	Pair/small group work, role play, drama	School nurse-led with client negotiation	To develop self-awareness, self-esteem and confidence
Physical and practical tasks	Scenarios, using condom demonstrators	Client-led with school nurse guidance	Development and attainment of skills
Provision of information	Leaflets, handouts, websites, posters	Client-led	To increase understanding further and allow access to relevant professionals/ agencies

what are the benefits in staying healthy and not taking risks? You might suggest that most children think smoking is uncool or most young people do not think unprotected sex is a good idea. Effective PSHE education, therefore, needs to start from where the child or young person is, and with an understanding of that position. It should promote self-esteem and motivation, foster emotional literacy, have positive expectations and be delivered within a continuous programme.

Valuing difference and diversity in PSHE

The UK is a multicultural society with children from widely differing backgrounds with diverse needs. The way in which schools and their pupils gain respect for a culturally diverse society is to ensure that PSHE education, alongside inclusion, is at the heart of the curriculum. Educational inclusion is a part of social inclusion, and its aim is to give every pupil, regardless of their background, the opportunity to fulfil their human potential. As discussed, the frameworks for PSHE education are important vehicles through which schools make concrete and explicit their provision. Healthy schools should address discrimination and inequality that exist in the school community (Kochar and Mitchell, 2002). Basic human rights mean that everyone has the right to an education and to feel safe within their community and powerful policy statements have been adopted by the international community following pressure from human rights activists including:

- *The Salamanca Statement* adopted by UNESCO in July 1994
- *The UN Convention on the Rights of the Child* (1989)
- *The UN Standard Rules on Equalisation* (1993)

Schools have a 'values framework' which sets out the overall philosophy of the school and its belief systems in relation to these policies. The *Sex and Relationship Education Guidance* (Department for Education and Employment [DfEE], 2000) emphasises that SRE should be sensitive to the range of values and beliefs, promoting self-discovery without the influence of the teacher's personal beliefs and attitudes. The key messages are:

- To promote debate and reflection in a safe environment.
- To encourage young people to formulate their own beliefs about individuals and groups of people, whilst not forcing particular attitudes on them.
- To promote anti-discriminatory attitudes.

Collaboration with school staff and parents is essential when planning and delivering potentially sensitive material to pupils, and respect for different value systems is crucial (SEF, 2004). School nurses also need to ensure that their own values and opinions do not influence the content of PSHE education or the responses to children and young people within it. A good PSHE lesson should contribute to the development of the learner without prejudice. As with all work that nurses do, anti-discriminatory practice is an essential part of the code of conduct (NMC, 2008).

Should school nurses have local PSHE education policies and what should they contain?

The Healthy Child Programme (HCP) (DH/DCSF, 2009b) affirms the need for all pupils to receive a comprehensive age-appropriate programme of PSHE to which school nurses can contribute. It also recognises that services may be delivered and staff deployed in different ways according to local circumstances and thus the HCP can be adapted to provide local guidance for school nurses. An example of how the school nursing service can plan to provide PSHE within the HCP is provided in Table 5.3.

The table specifically sets out the HCP core programme for PSHE for 11–19 years, providing guidance for the roles of different members of the school nursing team. In addition to the service outline of the HCP, a framework to provide further clarity around the role of school nurse teams and the practical day-to-day management of PSHE should also be developed locally. The protocol should be jointly endorsed by health and education and be evidence-based. It is a good idea to include a contract of agreement which can be completed with each school at the end of the academic year, setting out the plans for the next. This should outline what the school nurse is going to contribute to PSHE guidance, in line with the local HCP, and avoids *ad hoc* requests from schools. This can be renewed every year and be signed and dated by both parties. It is useful to have a working checklist (Table 5.4) to ensure that all areas of PSHE practice have been discussed and there is clear guidance for outside visitors.

An outline of the roles and responsibilities of both school nurses and school staff, such as in Table 5.5 is also a useful tool to include. The Sex Education Forum (SEF, 2011a) provides guidance on the roles and responsibilities of the school and the external visitor.

In PSHE, a school nurse's role is to complement teachers' work and not to replace the teacher's responsibility for covering PSHE. Having frameworks in place, as discussed, will help with continuity of practice and equity of service.

Table 5.3 Supporting schools in delivering PSHE.

Supporting schools and delivering PSHE education Key Stages 3 and 4

Core programme	Contact standard	Core content of contact	Action to be undertaken
Support schools in the delivery of health promotion To support ongoing Healthy Schools programmes	Specialist Community Public Health Nurse – School Nurse Band 6 and delegated to Community Staff Nurse Band 5 as appropriate	Meet with healthy schools/PSHE lead/school leadership/parents Discuss the defined responsibilities (see school nursing framework for PSHE) to plan and implement Contribution to policy and school development	Advising schools of the health needs of their population Contribute local/national health priorities Clarify the school nursing role Attend staff/governor meetings
		Provision of open access to school nursing for health promotion on a one-to-one basis and follow up after PSHE/SRE sessions	Provide a 'drop-in' type service (see related core programme) according to need.
		Provision of individual student appointments for health promotion on a one-to-one basis and follow up after PSHE/SRE sessions	Provide individual confidential one-to-one appointments to discuss issues (see related core programme)
		Provide up-to-date information on health services	Provide details of services to students in PSHE/SRE lessons, assemblies, stands (e.g. for No Smoking Day) or via displays. Brief staff in school who are involved with pastoral care and PSHE/SRE
Support schools in the delivery of PSHE/SRE for Key Stages 3, 4 and 5	Band 6	Meet with staff/governors/parents to plan a bespoke rolling programme to meet the needs of the school Confirm school nursing boundaries and responsibilities	Contact school to arrange a meeting in the summer term to plan for next academic year Complete contract (see school nursing framework for PSHE). School nursing service is unable to contribute without this. Also we are unable to provide one-off contributions that do not meet student learning needs

Table 5.3 (*continued*)

Supporting schools and delivering PSHE education Key Stages 3 and 4

Core programme	Contact standard	Core content of contact	Action to be undertaken
		Negotiation of school nursing's unique contribution to classroom education	Plan appropriate individual/team teaching to address issues with health expertise using checklist (see School nursing framework for PSHE) with staff Deliver programme in partnership with teachers Such as: KS 3: Healthy relationships How to access services KS3/4: Contraception, STIs, pregnancy and birth KS 4: Breast and testicular awareness KS4/5: Health advice in preparation for independent life, e.g. travel/university/work

Table 5.4 A working checklist.

.... **School checklist**
Date(s) of School Nursing contribution(s):
Specific areas of contribution by the School Nurse Team:
Agreed learning outcomes/objectives:
Lesson plans: (can be attached)
The school nurse knows/has received: ■ The relevant school policies such as; PSHE, SRE, drugs, bullying and confidentiality. ■ The school's whole PSHE programme outline, with a detailed copy of the relevant area they are being asked to contribute to. ■ Information about the groups they will be working with; age, sex, number, special needs etc. ■ A member of school staff will be present in the classroom during classroom PSHE and will be responsible for the behaviour of the pupils. ■ The school will provide agreed resources (e.g. condoms) as well as the appropriate space and equipment (e.g. computer, smart board, DVD player). ■ The length of the lesson, when to arrive, where to park, how to report arrival and arrangements for getting to the correct classroom.
Agreed evaluation mechanism and feedback to the school:

Table 5.5 School and school nursing team responsibilities with PSHE education.

School responsibilities	■ A commitment from the senior management team to support PSHE/SRE ■ To ensure Governors are involved within PSHE policies and provision within their school ■ Nominate a willing PSHE/SRE coordinator to provide and/or facilitate learning ■ Planning and delivery of statutory provision of PSHE and a policy agreed non-statutory provision of PSHE/SRE ■ Identify and involve outside agencies to provide unique and appropriate contributions ■ Provide suitable environment for individual health interventions (one to ones) and open access service such as school nurse drop-in and health zones ■ Provide suitable environment for school nurse team to deliver PSHE, including provision of resources (e.g. white boards, computers) ■ Classroom management and student discipline during sessions ■ Understand that the contribution of the school nurse team is governed by their mandatory responsibilities. Therefore agreed contribution must always reflect that ■ Organise and agree contribution of school nurse team annually and complete contract in the summer term which precedes the academic year which the contract addresses
School and school nursing team responsibilities	■ Policy development ■ Planning and consultation with staff, parents and pupils ■ Access to relevant training ■ Information in regards to up to date and new resources ■ Development of increased access to health services on site as appropriate e.g. health zone ■ Awareness of the difference and diversity within PSHE/SRE ■ Ensuring effective evaluation of PSHE/SRE and basing future planning upon this ■ Information giving, e.g. local health services ■ Parent meetings addressing PSHE/SRE *(Note that many school nursing teams do not work past 5 p.m.; therefore meetings where you require school nursing support should be arranged during the daytime)*
School nursing team responsibilities	■ Updating school staff delivering PSHE/SRE on local health services and needs within the local community ■ Raising awareness of the health needs of pupils ■ Negotiating unique contribution to whole school PSHE/SRE within framework ■ Individual health interviews/one-to-ones, including (as appropriate) individual education relating to PSHE/SRE ■ Open access service for both parents and pupils including as appropriate individual education relating to PSHE/SRE ■ Referral/signposting ■ Provision of drop-in service for Key Stages 3, 4 and 5, including student visits to drop-in/health zone as part of pre-planned programme if applicable ■ Be aware of and work within the school's policies **School nursing teams cannot offer**: isolated planning or *ad hoc* delivery of PSHE to groups of pupils that do not meet a specific identified need or PSHE without the completion of the contract

Planning a PSHE session

When planning and delivering PSHE it is important to liaise with:

- Governors and head teachers:
    - To make sure the sessions are within the remit of the school policies
    - To ensure school nurses are aware of the background of the pupils and the ethos of the school, including religion, culture and ethnicity
- Class teacher and PSHE leads:
  Pre-lesson:
    - To reaffirm role clarity and plan team-teaching approach if appropriate
    - To ensure lessons are in line with pupils' needs
    - To gain information regarding previous lessons taught
    - To provide the context within which school nurse sessions are taking place. Teachers are aware of the children's knowledge concerning the subject(s) covered, and this will help with the preparation of possible inappropriate or diverse questioning
    - To understand the curriculum objectives. School nurses must not be afraid to ask the teacher advice on how they think the lesson should be delivered
    - To provide advice on the academic ability of the class as well as the size and age to assist the choice of teaching methods to support inclusion
    - To ensure the presence of a classroom teacher during the session to 'control' the class
  Post-lesson:
    - To provide feedback regarding the lessons
    - To encourage continuity in learning through assessment of what further work needs to be done
- Parents and carers
    - To provide an arena for discussion of PSHE particularly around SRE, making sure parents are aware of the input being given at school
    - So they can ask the school nurse about their specific contribution
    - To enable them to make an informed decision as to whether they want to remove their child from the non-statutory SRE part of the curriculum
    - To promote the role of the school nurse further
- Pupils:
    - To know what the pupils themselves want from a lesson. This can be done through the evaluation of previous lessons or using a pre-session questionnaire or pre-session class visit

- To see whether they have any particular wishes for the lesson, e.g. single-sex lessons.
- To gather ideas of what they feel would be beneficial for them to learn
- To start to develop/further develop school nurse–pupil relationships

By giving children an active role they can develop a sense of ownership of their learning. This leads to empowerment, thus allowing them to make valuable contributions and take part in decision-making regarding their health. Education related to values is best when it involves all members of the learning community – teachers, students and non-teaching staff, as well as parents, in a whole school approach (DfES, 2004).

Delivering PHSE education

Schools vary widely in their models of PSHE delivery. This is true particularly within secondary education, as it is often a marginalised subject due to time constraints caused by the statutory curriculum. Modes of delivery include:

- **Dedicated PSHE teachers** planning and providing full programmes of regular weekly timetabled PSHE lessons is the ideal. They have the skills and confidence to teach the subject and the time to organise specific external visitors.
- **Class teachers or form tutors** are the most common choice by schools for delivering PSHE education. However, studies show that teachers have a lack of appropriate training as well as preparatory time in order to deliver effective sessions (St Leger, 2000). PSHE carried out by class/form tutors is more likely to be *ad hoc* and short in length, as many use the sessions for other things, which is not ideal (Ofsted, 2010).
- **PSHE days** are where schools collapse the usual timetable to allow for PSHE 'Theme Days'. This can happen from once a year to up to twice a term. Schools think that they are providing memorable days that pupils will enjoy and therefore keep in mind what is taught. However, it is recognised that pupils do not always respond well to such days, as they need time to process what is taught and revisit their learning. They are useful in conjunction with other regular PSHE sessions.
- **Peer education** is where older pupils deliver either part of or whole PSHE lessons to their younger peers. The thought behind peer education is that young people influence each other's attitudes and behaviours. Through PSHE, young people can act as credible role models for their younger peers and hopefully lead them to engage in healthy behaviours. Kim and Free's (2008) systematic

review showed that there is little evidence for the benefits of peer education, but that children and young people often rate it highly as it is presented at their level and in their language. It is also worth noting that research indicates that peer education is evaluated well by black and ethnic minority groups (Emmerson, 2011).

- **Theatre in education** is where an educational topic or debate is presented as a show or play, usually by a visiting theatre company. There are a number of companies in the UK that specialise in producing theatre to be performed in schools, but it is a resource that not all schools can afford. Mages *et al.* (2007) found that young people could identify with the characters and talk about them and their choices. This enabled them to discuss sensitive topics such as sexual health with more confidence, as it wasn't personal to them and this helped them to feel safe. Theatre in education can be really enjoyable, and therefore memorable, for pupils.

Once the initial planning has been undertaken and the context for the delivery of the PSHE sessions has been determined school nurses then need to set out the aims and outcomes for their sessions (see Chapter 2). An example of a lesson plan is in Table 5.6.

Active learning

This approach to learning should promote active engagement of the pupils in the learning process. In practice, this way of learning lends itself mostly to group work, which is different from the more formal teaching in most lessons. Effective group work using active learning techniques is particularly suited to PSHE as it provides the following benefits:

- It can be used with pupils of all ages and abilities, enabling everyone to participate from different starting points, ensuring everyone is valued.
- Pupil's self-esteem can be enhanced, as they realise that it is OK to make mistakes in smaller groups.
- Views and opinions can be explored rather than prescribed as fixed. Different lifestyles, cultures, values and beliefs are acknowledged and respected.
- Pupils are more active in their own learning and this can increase their energy levels and interest in the subject, keeping them engaged and motivated.
- The variety of learning experiences introduces an element of fun and helps them to enjoy their learning.

Table 5.6 An example of a detailed girls' puberty lesson.

Date:	School: Anywhere Junior School
Time:	Key stage: 2 Year: 5 and 6 Class: 30 girls and carers
	Pupils with SEN and provision: 0

Name of school nurse:

Previous learning in the area and context:
National Curriculum – Key Stage 2: Rolling PSHE knowledge, skills and understanding and science programme. Further joint SRE to be covered in Year 6.

Intended learning outcomes:
Each child will be encouraged:
1. To make a positive contribution and have the opportunity to begin to develop confidence in talking, listening and thinking about growing up.
2. To understand that they are growing/changing or that they will grow/change and that it happens at different times for different people.
3. To understand what these changes are (physical and emotional) and how they may affect them.
4. To understand that it is a normal life process.
5. To be able to name parts of the reproductive system using correct biological terminology.
6. To look at and discuss sanitary protection.
7. To identify their mother or another adult as point of contact that they can speak to regarding issues around puberty.

Each mother/carer/friend will:
1. Be included in maintaining a climate of trust and mutual respect between all those involved.
2. Be encouraged to make a positive contribution.
3. Be approachable, supportive and a person their child can trust.
4. Come away with ideas about how to talk their child about puberty, sex and relationships.

Materials/resources:
Puberty DVD
PowerPoint demonstration
Roller coaster resource pack – 'monthly match game'
Quiz sheets and 'Check out the Changes' sheets
Display boards for leaflet display and reproductive system posters
Examples of sanitary protection
Access to a board/large piece of paper and a pen
'Ask it basket' for anonymous questions for when I return next week
Worksheets for homework
Evaluation forms for teachers, parents/carers and pupils
Leaflets for the girls on puberty and hygiene
Leaflets for the parents/carers for themselves and also some to share with the girls at a later date

Table 5.6 (*continued*)

Main teaching and learning strategies:
Introduction and ground rules discussion – whole-class structured group work
Pair work with the quiz – willingness to work with one another cooperatively and encouraging children who may feel isolated within the class to participate
Group work – discussion of changes in puberty and individual writing to aid learning
Looking at a PowerPoint demonstration
Watching a short excerpt from a DVD
Small group work with parents/carers
Inclusion/differentiation strategies:
Negotiation of ground rules
Ensuring all pupils are given equal speaking time and those not wishing to contribute and not pressurised to do so
Different learning needs are identified and catered for
Opportunity for girls to look at sanitary protection and talk to facilitator away from parent/carer
Assessment strategies:
Verbal responses from the children
Observation during the session
Knowledge level assessed form the completed worksheets post session
Evaluations from the teaching staff and pupils
Discussion with the teachers for future adaption if required

Session plan – activities and approximate timings

Time	Community nurse's activity	Pupils' activity
15:30	Introduce self to group and aims of the session	Sit in whole group and listen
15:35	Negotiate ground rules and emphasise their importance. Display using PowerPoint	Listen to ground rules and participate as a group to add on any which they feel are appropriate
15:40	Girls to complete quiz together in pairs, in order for facilitator to assess prior knowledge	Pair work
15:45	Using the quiz answers as pointers to highlight the changes that occur in puberty. Use PowerPoint. Pupils to make their own notes on 'body sheets' if they wish	Group discussion with pupils, carers and facilitator Individual note taking if the girls wish too
15:55	Encourage a quick discussion on what coping mechanisms they might use when they are going through a variety of feelings	Group discussion with both pupils and carers to participate and confer with one another. Individuals to feedback their ideas

Table 5.6 (*continued*)

Time	Community nurse's activity	Pupils' activity
16:00	Watch DVD	Group watching and listening
16:05	Talk about menstruation in more detail, use posters	Group listening and asking of relevant questions. Playing game 'monthly match' in small groups
16:15	Show and explain sanitary protection and the importance of keeping healthy. Show products and PowerPoint	Group listening and asking relevant questions
16:25	Sum up the session. Ask the pupils and carers if they have any final questions Encourage parents to pick up information and fill in an evaluation	Encourage individual responses Individual carer evaluation completion and possible carer discussion
16:30	Encourage girls to look at sanitary products, pick up leaflets and discuss any concerns or questions that they might have. Explain about the 'ask it basket' for their questions, homework worksheets and evaluations	Small group discussion. Completion of worksheets and evaluations by pupils at a later date.

- It encourages and improves pupils social and communication skills, as they are less dependent on the adult teaching for their learning, and are engaging in collaborative work with their peers (Ainsworth, 2009).
- It provides a supportive and safe context for personal reflection, growth and experimentation. They can develop core life skills, such as empathy, decision-making and listening.

Sessions should use a mixture of different teaching methods: DVD, PowerPoint presentations, debates, small and large group discussions, quizzes/questionnaires and scenarios can all be used to provoke thought and initiate the formation of opinions. Younger children particularly enjoy the freedom of circle time and role play and this can be used to encourage them to share their thoughts and feelings, as everyone should have the opportunity to be heard.

Useful activities include:

■ **Trigger material**

– *Stories, poems, pictures, drawings and photographs* – these can all be used to introduce subjects leading to brain storming, discussion and/or debate. This is appropriate for all key stages.

– *Quizzes and questionnaires* – these can either be done in pairs or in larger groups, and allow the school nurse to identify pupils' knowledge and understanding of a topic. Suitable for all ages, but ensure they are quite short and fun to do.

– *Question boxes* – pupils put anonymous questions into a box about the topic being taught which are then answered by the school nurse at a given point. This is usually most appropriate at the end of a lesson and allows pupils to ask questions about sensitive subjects that they may not feel able to do in front of their peers, such as puberty in Key Stage 2 and sex and relationships in Key Stages 3 and 4.

– *Puppets* – these can be bought or homemade by cutting out pictures from magazines or drawing figures. Puppets can be used to tell a story or as a basis for discussion for sensitive issues and are most suited to Key Stage 1 and 2. Issues such as bullying, relationships, good touch and bad touch can be addressed. Red Riding Hood puppets can be useful to teach protective behaviours.

– *Diamond Nines* – statements are placed on nine individual pieces of paper. Pupils are divided into groups, given a set of statements and asked to discuss and place the statements in order of priority in a diamond shape: one at the top, two on the next line, three in the middle, two below and one at the bottom. This activity is most suited to Key Stage 2 and above and can involve such things as the most important qualities of a healthy relationship or the most harmful drugs. This activity can also be used with one or two blank statements, allowing pupils to add their own ideas.

– *Listening exercises* – these can include listening to a song, a story, a poem or someone talking about a subject. They could also include pair work involving one pupil listening while the other speaks. Roles can then be swapped and information fed back if appropriate. Appropriate for Key Stage 2 and above and can be used for a variety of subjects; for example: how do you feel about growing up?

– *Graffiti sheets* – sheets of paper are placed around the room with different headings/questions on each. Pupils move around the room and write simple responses on the sheets. Useful for Key Stage 3 and above and can be used for a wide range of PSHE topics. A simple idea is to write different drug names on each piece of paper: pupils then write anything they know about each one.

■ **Discussion and debates**

- *Open questioning* – asking pupils open-ended questions about a particular subject achieves a wider range of responses and initiates further discussion. In order to involve the whole class it may be necessary to break pupils into smaller groups.

- *Discussion groups* – all types of groups work: pairs, fours, splitting the class into quarters or half. Separate gender groups may be appropriate for sensitive topics. Pupils get to share their ideas and experiences, as well as practising such skills as speaking, listening and cooperation.

- *Reporting back* – after a smaller group discussion or other task, each group is asked to share what they have talked about to the rest of the class.

- *Circle time* – pupils sit in a circle and pass round an item such as a teddy. With the introduction of a statement such as 'I am good at...', the item gets passed round the circle and those who want to contribute do so when they are holding the 'teddy'. Those who do not want to speak do not have to, but are able to contribute by passing the item to the next person. This is particularly suitable for Key Stage 1 pupils.

- *Continuums* – this involves pupils physically placing themselves along a line that represents their view point on a particular subject. Each end of the line represents an opposite opinion, for example Agree/Disagree, Right/Wrong, Like/Dislike. The aim is to hear people's views and the reasons for them, facilitating discussion. This will be most successful with later Key Stage 2 (years 5 and 6) and above. This idea can also be used with other types of continuum, particularly in Key Stages 3 and 4; for example pupils physically placing themselves, on a line that represents ages 10 to 60, where they think it's the right age to start having sex, to have a baby etc.

- *Fish bowl discussion* – a small circle of chairs are placed together within a larger circle. The majority of the class sits in the outer circle, with a few sitting on the chairs in the middle, ensuring that at least one of these inner chairs is empty. A topic is introduced and only the pupils in the inner circle can discuss it. Others can move in and out of the circle to join or leave the debate as they wish. Great for Key Stage 3 and above.

- *Carousels/standpoint talking* – Pupils sit in two circles which face each other. The group is given a statement which they have to discuss, one circle being 'for' and the other 'against'. They then debate with the person in front of them. After a given period of time move the outer circle on two places. The process can be repeated as many times as necessary and the circles can also change their 'stance'. This is based on the speed dating idea, allowing the development of speaking, listening and refection skills. Again, this is more suitable for older pupils.

■ **Distancing techniques**
- *Case studies* – pupils are introduced and invited to think about and respond to a character and their situation or dilemma. It is useful as a school nurse to be up to date with the TV soap storylines, as many young people follow these programmes. It can be useful in Key Stages 3 and 4 PSHE to refer to these, discussing the course of action by certain characters or empathising and identifying with certain situations.
- *Role play, drama and scenarios* – these involve pupils using their imagination to take on the role of other characters to discuss certain topics or scenarios. It will encourage young people to view situations from someone else's viewpoint. An example would be that boys take on the role of a pregnant teenager and the girls the father.

■ **Media**
- *Videos/DVDs, TV programmes, web pages, CD-ROMs, PowerPoint presentations, interactive white boards* – technology allows a huge range of opportunities to engage young people in a medium that they are familiar with.
- *Analysis* – use of reflection on certain material such as magazines, newspapers or TV advertisements, campaigns and articles. It has been particularly useful to create discussion around celebrity images where young people are influenced by body image and what they see as perfection.
- *Current issues in the press/national awareness days* – these are useful areas for discussion.

Practical tips for teaching PSHE
■ Rehearse the planned session for timings and content in advance.
■ Dressing in layers will enable adjustment of clothing to the temperature of the room and allow the school nurse to remain comfortable. Take water with you as nerves can give you a dry mouth.
■ Follow school guidelines on working in the classroom.
■ Set up the room according to how the session is going to run, for example if you are using circles of chairs.

- Make sure a teacher is with you in the classroom.
- Preferably be there to 'meet and greet' the pupils (be early, not late).
- Ask the teacher to introduce you.
- Explain who you are and your role and how you expect them to behave.
- Explain what the session involves and what they will be expected to do.
- Establish ground rules and write them down, for example:
    - Listen to others and wait your turn.
    - Be mature; use correct terminology.
    - Show respect and try to understand one another's opinions.
    - Ask questions; no question is a silly question.
    - No personal questions will be asked or answered.
    - Maintain confidentiality: 'What is said in this room stays in this room'.

    The ground rules should be 'dos' rather than 'don'ts' to enhance a positive atmosphere. School nurses should not be afraid to stop the lesson in order to remind pupils of the rules if they feel they are not being followed. If they are written or displayed throughout the lesson they can be referred to as needed.
- Take care not to disclose personal information and discourage others from doing so. If you run a drop-in, mention this for young people to access if they have concerns about anything that is raised.
- Follow child protection procedures if there is a disclosure by a pupil in the classroom.
- Use an icebreaker if necessary and if you have time. Pupils may know each other but not you.
- Use the class teacher to support you in managing the class. Be clear with them beforehand what your expectation of them is.
- If you are doing group work, ensure that everyone understands what is expected of them and keep the groups to time.
- While the pupils are working on tasks which involve discussion in groups it is a good idea to walk slowly around the room and listen to what is being said. It is important not to get too close and interrupt their discussions, but to let them have the freedom to explore the subject. School nurses should only intervene if they are concerned that the pupils do not seem to understand the activity or seem to be discussing incorrect information. If pupils are having difficulty or are having a particularly heated discussion the school nurse can join in the group and ask open-ended questions such as 'Why do you think that?' or 'Are they right or wrong?' to help control and guide them (Ainsworth, 2009).

■ Throughout the lesson, continual assessment by observing pupil participation and listening to their ideas and responses will ensure that the information given and the activities used are being understood. Do not be afraid to change or modify lesson plans if needed.

■ Make sure that you leave the session with at least one key message that you wanted to get across.

Suggestions for the end of a session

■ *Closing rounds* – good sentence ideas for a round are 'I have learnt that...' and 'I was surprised that...'. For Key Stage 1 and 2 pupils it can be useful to have an object such as a teddy that they can pass round the group; whoever has the teddy identifies whose turn it is to finish the sentence.

■ *Advice to others* – for example, if the school nurse was teaching about sexually transmitted infections the last activity of the lesson could be to ask the group 'What advice would you give to someone who thinks they might be at risk of contracting an STI?'. Answers can be written on the board and be used to summarise the main points of the lesson (PSHE Association, 2010).

■ *Four word/phrase build/'snowballing'* – pupils are asked to think on their own of four words or phrases that are the key messages to take away from the lesson. Each pupil then joins with another, discusses and agrees four from their eight. They then join with another pair and do the same; this continues until the class has come to a final conclusive four words/phrases.

■ *Alien* – this activity is more suited to Key Stage 2 and 3 pupils. Pupils are told that they have to imagine that an alien has come to earth and has no knowledge about the subject being taught. How will they describe it to the alien? A list of questions that the alien may ask could be provided. For example for the subject of drugs: What are they? What do they look like? What are they used for? Who uses them? Why?

■ *Draw and write* – this task involves asking pupils to draw or write or both, dependent on pupil age and ability, in response to a question or statement such as: 'What are the effects of drug use?', 'What is a healthy diet?' or 'Three things you know about smoking' (Wetton and Williams, 2000).

Evaluating the session

■ *Pupil perspective (be aware of age appropriateness)*
  – Sticky notes on a board.
  – A brief questionnaire, either at the end of the session or later. This will need to be age appropriate, using pictures for young children or more

complex questions for older children. You can customise questionnaires according to the age and abilities of the group. It is good practice to discuss this with the teacher beforehand.

- Focus groups – a more detailed way of evaluating sessions is to ask pupils directly in smaller groups. This is useful if the school nurse is on a spiral curriculum throughout the school year.

■ *Teacher perspective* – evaluation by teaching staff will enable the school nurse to identify what was done well and what changes need to be made for future lessons. Again, this could be done formally though a written questionnaire or informally by a conversation post-lesson or asking the teacher to provide some feedback via email.

■ *Parental perspective* – if the parents were invited to the lesson (e.g. a puberty lesson for both girls and their parents), getting the parents' feedback is also useful. They can provide interesting information regarding the provision by the school for PSHE, how useful they found lesson, how useful they think their child found it, whether it was enjoyable and what could be improved. This can be done by direct questioning, questionnaires or suggestion boxes.

■ *Peer observations* – it is useful from time to time for school nurses to observe each other in PSHE work. This will give valuable insight into performance and help avoid becoming entrenched in one way of presenting information.

As with all types of assessment and evaluation it is important not to look at each one in isolation but to see how they feed in to each other and also how they compare with the school nurse's own reflections of the lesson. Useful questions for the school nurse to ask herself are:

■ Were the lesson objectives achieved?
■ Were the pupils engaged? Were boys and girls equally engaged? Was anyone excluded?
■ Did they work on all the tasks set? If not, why not?
■ Did they answer my questions?
■ Were they able to ask their own?
■ What did and didn't work well? What could I do differently? (Sex Education Forum, 2005a).

How should school nurses work with pupils who have special educational needs or learning difficulties?

School nurses will need to consider the needs of children and young people with special educational needs both in mainstream and in specialised schools. It is important to be inclusive in sessions and this will require planning with school staff according to need. Any adaptation of the sessions should be carefully considered to avoid alienating anyone in the classroom. In some cases, discussions with parents may also be appropriate. Depending on the difficulty, there may be learning support assistants available to help in the session. There should be recognition that the school nurse may not be the most appropriate person to deliver information, but they can provide help with the content if needed.

Some examples of children with special needs:

- Pupils with speech, language and communication difficulties may need some support to understand and share feelings. School nurses could use techniques such as visual aids including pictures, stories, puppets and role play to teach these aspects (The Communication Trust, 2009).
- Pupils with social communication disorders such as autism and Asperger's may require logical teaching about themes such as feelings. Care should be taken about the language you use to ensure that there is no ambiguity. Stories may be useful, with the inclusion of symbols or pictures to show facial expressions and social interactions (Staffordshire County Council, 2008).
- For children and young people with difficulties in concentration and/or behavioural issues such as attention deficit and/or hyperactive disorders, physical activities may be more appropriate. Or working with smaller groups on shorter activities with possible rest breaks (Training and Development Agency for Schools, 2009).

Sex and Relationships Education (SRE)

A key role for school nurses is their contribution to sex and relationships education (SRE). They have expert knowledge about sexual health and they are trusted adults for young people. SRE should provide children and young people with the skills and knowledge to develop fulfilling, healthy, safe relationships and to handle, with confidence, their transition into adulthood (Family Planning Association [FPA], 2011). This includes exploring issues around appropriate, loving relationships and recognising abusive situations (see Chapter 4). However, SRE remains variable across the country, school health teams are stretched and pressure for academic achievement means that SRE can be a neglected area. Anecdotal evidence, however, suggests that where school nurses have been withdrawn from SRE there has been a rise in teenage pregnancy in individual schools. Further evidence is needed in this respect to demonstrate a need.

The SRE curriculum teaches three main elements:

- **Attitudes and values** – respect for self and others, morality, and recognising the benefit of stable, loving relationships and family life. This should also include appropriate and inappropriate relationships.
- **Personal and social skills** – negotiation skills, building confidence and self-esteem, developing empathy, sensitivity and making healthy and safe choices.
- **Knowledge and understanding** – physical and emotional development, puberty, sexuality, reproduction, contraception, STIs, unplanned pregnancy, abortion and reasons for delaying sexual activity, as well as where local and national sexual health resources and services can be found.

Some of this is compulsory within the science curriculum:

- **Key stages 1 and 2**: biological aspects, names of sexual organs, puberty
- **Key stages 3 and 4**: human reproduction and diseases associated with sexual health

Other SRE is at the discretion of the school in consultation with governors and parents. The government's SRE guidance (DfEE, 2000) provides policy and practice direction for schools and is supported in legislation by the Learning and Skills Act (HMSO, 2000):

- School governing bodies must decide what SRE within PSHE education will be included in the curriculum.
- All policies should be made in consultation with parents, pupils, teachers and governors.
- All schools must ensure that the needs of all pupils are met regardless of culture, ethnicity, religion or sexual orientation, including those with particular needs.
- There should be an emphasis on the three main elements: attitudes and values; personal and social skills; and knowledge and understanding.
- Appropriate activities should be used to meet the needs of both boys and young men and girls and young women.
- Primary SRE should ensure that pupils know about puberty before it starts.
- SRE should not be taught in isolation but be firmly rooted within planned PSHE education delivery.

The current legal status of SRE within academies and free schools differs. They are not required to have an up-to-date SRE policy or teach SRE, unlike state-maintained schools (SEF, 2011a). It is important for school nurses to be aware of this, as the number of academies is increasing throughout England and this could affect what they will contribute to and provide from one school to the next.

In 2010 guidance was updated for schools on SRE (DCSF, 2010; NICE, 2010). These updates reflected the recognition for good quality SRE that equips children and young people not just with information and knowledge, but also with the skills they need to form healthy and positive relationships. It describes effective SRE as ensuring that children grow up to enjoy positive and loving relationships, and to be informed about and be comfortable with puberty, sexual activity and health, as well as being emotionally secure. There is also emphasis on being safe, given the growing risks of grooming behaviour both via the internet and also in the community. The Schools White Paper (DE, 2010) made clear the coalition government's intention to review all existing guidance, including SRE, with the aim of simplification and reformation.

How do children and young people feel about SRE?

Many surveys have been conducted and they demonstrate similar findings: that many young people have inadequate sexual health knowledge. For years, children and young people have stated that SRE is often 'too late, too little and too biological' (Emmerson, 2011, p. 218). Many young people either find SRE unhelpful or have not received any SRE at all (Chamberlain *et al.*, 2010). Many say it is poorly delivered and insufficiently supported by both written materials and opportunities to get further advice (FPA, 2007). In one survey of young people, 73% felt it should be taught earlier and over 60% of males and females reported not being taught anything about personal relationships (UK Youth Parliament, 2007). In another, 75% of respondents felt that how to resist peer pressure was insufficiently covered and half stated that contraception was inadequately taught (DfES, 2007). Westwood and Mullan (2006) found that significant numbers of Year 10 pupils lacked knowledge about STIs. Thirty-one per cent did not know what chlamydia was and 56% did not know that syphilis was an STI. This is important evidence for school nurses, justifying the provision of their services to the commissioners within public health.

How do parents feel about SRE and what is their role?

Research indicates that most parents feel that school-based SRE is beneficial for their children (SEF, 2011a) and that it should cover relationships and emotional aspects, as well as the biological facts (Durex *et al.*, 2010). Some parents have criticised the fact that the provision of SRE differs between schools and that it should be provided in more depth and earlier (Durex *et al.*, 2010). Others are resistant to any information being given outside the family.

Parents see school and themselves as the two main sources of SRE (Sherbert Research, 2009). Children and young people state that parents are an important source of learning about sex and relationships and their preferred choice of educator (SEF, 2008). School nursing confirms that many young people feel unsupported by their parents or express anxiety at sharing concerns with parents or professionals regarding their sexual health (Hayward, 2011). Research also shows that the young people at greatest risk of pregnancy or contracting STIs are the least likely to access mainstream services (Brook, 2008).

A UK study identified that parents do have the skills to educate their children in these matters (Walker, 2001) and school nurses have the expertise to harness these skills in order to empower parents in encouraging their children to make healthy and safe choices.

Key points about encouraging parents to talk to their children

- Open and honest communication with parents to engage them in the process and content of SRE. Provide a forum for parents to meet the school nurse and teachers. Often, reassurance for parents is crucial.
- Encourage parents to discuss the content of the sessions with their children at home.
- The invitation to parents/guardians to specific single-sex puberty sessions (mother and daughter or father and son evenings, for example) is still a popular idea used by some Key Stage 2 teachers.
- The provision of, or signposting to, useful resources for parents such as those produced by the Sex Education Forum is welcomed by most. Other publishers also produce excellent resources for stimulating discussion.
- Providing parents with the skills and knowledge to talk to their children about growing up through a parenting programme is useful.
- Help to facilitate better communication between young people and their parents. As most children and young people identify their parents as being the most preferred person to learn about sex and relationships from, it could be argued that school nurses should prioritise this aspect of their SRE role. Research shows that young people who are able to talk honestly to their parents about sex and relationships are less likely to engage in risky behaviours (FPA, 2011).

Encouraging abstinence

There has been recent debate around teaching abstinence, which has been a common phenomenon in the USA in recent years. Not all abstinence education is the same, but it has the same basic underlying principle: that there are health, social and emotional benefits to avoiding sex before marriage. Some abstinence programmes also omit facts pertaining to safer sex, contraception or healthy sexuality with the view that it is better not to have sex before marriage. It is important for school nurses to be aware that these programmes may not prepare young people effectively or realistically about sex and could lead them to be secretive about their sexual activity. Young people may also feel an emotional consequence of being unable to abstain (Hayward, 2011). Evaluation of this type of SRE programme is not optimistic: there is no robust or conclusive evidence that instilling positive attitudes about abstinence either prevents teenage sexual activity or protects them from its consequences (Bennett and Assefi, 2005; Underhill *et al.*, 2007). However, encouraging loving and supportive relationships is a very important part of SRE and should be considered fundamental.

Issues and topics in SRE

Gender differences and needs

- An understanding of gender differences should underpin all SRE (FPA, 2011).
- Single-sex sessions can considerably ease pupils concerns and help them to feel safer and less embarrassed to discuss specific gender-related issues.
- Single-sex puberty lessons allow children to be more open about how they feel about growing up and becoming an adult. These should be backed up by sessions with both boys and girls together so that they learn about each other's development (SEF, 2000, 2006).
- Secondary pupils may want some single-sex lessons where they can have a more comfortable discussion around such issues as contraception and the mechanics of sex. It is important to try to provide these when needed; using break times is a possibility if there isn't space in the timetable.
- There may be gender differences in attitudes regarding relationships and sexual activity. Young women may be more likely to associate emotional attachment with sex, whereas young men may focus more on the physical pleasure of sexual activity and be more competitive (FPA, 2007). School nurses need to be able to facilitate discussion around these issues so that young people are aware of these potential differences and develop the same knowledge of the link between emotions, relationships and sexual activity.
- School nurse practice indicates that, generally, boys do not access health professionals or talk to their parents about sexual health as often as girls do. It is, therefore, an important consideration in the planning of SRE to ensure that boys' needs are met as effectively as those of girls (Hayward, 2011).

Primary school SRE (all need to be age appropriate)

- Recognising and communicating feelings.
- Naming parts of the body, including reproductive organs.
- Understanding gender differences.
- Understanding puberty prior to starting it.
- Exploring the nature of relationships and sexuality.
- Building confidence, self-esteem and self-worth. Learning to say no and developing negotiating skills.
- Risky behaviours and sexual exploitation – consideration of the safe use of the internet. It is important that parents are aware of what young children are accessing via the internet.

Secondary school SRE

As well as building on the above topics the following topics are covered:

- **Contraception:**
  - Assertiveness skills for negotiating relationships, contraceptive use and accessing services.
  - The importance of choosing a method/s that protect against both pregnancy and STIs.
  - How to use, and the importance of using, methods correctly and consistently, in particular the contraceptive pill and the condom.
  - The benefits of long-acting reversible contraception (LARC) for young people.
  - Ensuring all myths surrounding condom use are discussed, and all young people are able to practise placing a condom on a demonstrator if they so wish.
  - What emergency contraception is and how it should be used.
  - How and where to get both relevant advice and contraception, including free condoms and emergency contraception in the local area.
  - That all children and young people are entitled to confidential advice with regard to sexual health from any health professional, including the school nurse.
- **Sexually transmitted infections:**
  - Assertiveness skills for negotiating relationships, contraceptive use and accessing services.
  - Clarification of their knowledge of STIs, HIV and AIDS: how they are spread, what activities are the most risky and how to reduce the risk.

- That some STIs do not have obvious symptoms or may be symptomless, that you cannot always tell if you or your partner has one, and that some have severe long-term consequences for health.
- Ensuring that all biological and social myths surrounding STIs, especially HIV and AIDS, are discussed.
- How the use of barriers such as male and female condoms and dental dams will help prevent the transmission of some STIs during both heterosexual and homosexual activities.
- Ensuring all myths surrounding condom use are discussed, and all young people are able to have a go at practising placing a condom on a demonstrator if they so wish.
- That sexually active people should access STI testing after they have had unprotected sex, in-between partners as well as getting in the habit of having a 'once a year' check-up. Normalising this check-up by comparing it to optician and dental check-ups will help pupils to understand this concept.
- What STI testing involves and where it can be accessed.
- How negative attitudes and social stigma can affect people with HIV and AIDS and ensuring that stereotypes are challenged.

■ **Teenage pregnancy and abortion**:
- Revisiting the science of reproduction in order to dispel myths.
- Awareness of choices and appropriate services.
- Teaching young people about abortion means they can explore fully the issues of unintended pregnancy and are then better placed both to avoid unintended pregnancy in the first place, and to manage it should it ever become a reality (DH, 2001).
- Pregnancy should also be highlighted as a positive as well as a negative – young people are potential parents.

■ **Sexuality**:
- There are specific concerns from young people themselves that SRE is heavily focused on heterosexual relationships and that elements are irrelevant for homosexual young people (FPA, 2007). Thus, for many young people who identify themselves as being lesbian, gay or bisexual (LGB), SRE can lead to them feeling marginalised, unsupported and misunderstood.
- Some schools still remain confused over section 28, part of the Local Government Act 1988 (HMSO, 1988), which stated that a local authority shall not intentionally promote homosexuality or publish material with

the intention of promoting homosexuality. Even though it never applied to schools and has now been repealed, teachers remain in doubt over what they can and can't say about sexuality within SRE lessons. Discussing homosexuality does not promote it.

–   School nurses need to challenge any homophobic behaviour or remarks made within SRE (SEF, 2005b). It needs to be tackled in a way that helps young people to identify why it is unacceptable and how it may be hurtful. The use of ground rules will enable this to be a normal part of SRE lessons. This consistently drives forward the message that discrimination is not acceptable.

PSHE educational resources

It is common for teachers to use national government-approved resources, such as the social and emotional aspects of learning (SEAL), or well-known mass-produced resources such as the *Living and Growing* DVD series produced by Channel 4. Many local authorities produce their own, or adapt or signpost teachers to relevant PSHE education materials. A list of possible resources is provided at the end of this chapter.

Helpful criteria for selecting resources

- Does it meet the needs of the statutory and non-statutory curriculum and learning outcomes you have been asked to contribute to?
- Does it suggest how it can be linked to other lessons or how the ideas can be developed on? Could it be used as part of a spiral-type curriculum?
- Does it meet the needs of the pupils in terms of the required knowledge, understanding, ability and attitudes?
- Is the resource inclusive of all? (That is, not racist, sexist, stereotypical or homophobic, but takes all circumstances into consideration including all religious, cultural, social and financial backgrounds.)
- Is the resource able to be adapted for different individual or groups of pupils, e.g. single-sex, disability, special needs or the vulnerable?
- Does the resource reflect the ethos of the school you are going to be using it in and fit within their PSHE policy?
- Does it include positive images of children and young people?
- Does it contain active learning methods, encouraging the development and reflection of knowledge, skills, attitudes and values?

Both the PSHE Association and the Sex Education Forum have produced useful guidance for helping practitioners select appropriate PSHE resources.

Conclusion

The first ever child health strategy was seen as a signal in the prioritising of service improvement enabling effective child-centred public health. The transfer of the responsibility of public health to Local Authorities offers an opportunity to develop a more targeted and integrated approach to PSHE education. Both public health and children's service directors will work together, with the knowledge of local data informing commissioning. It is hoped that this time the good intentions are implemented and funding is provided so that service quality can be improved, allowing the UK to be among the better, rather than the worst, countries in terms of young people's health and wellbeing.

For school nurses, work within the public health framework is made up of a wide range of activities, including health promotion, protection and prevention, as well as public health policy and individual and community empowerment. School nurses work with individual children, families, specific class/year groups and whole school communities to promote health. SRE is a lifelong learning process of acquiring information, developing skills and forming positive beliefs and attitudes about sex, sexuality, relationships and feelings. For school nurses, effective SRE can make a significant contribution to the development of the personal skills needed by young people if they are to establish and maintain relationships. It also enables young people to make responsible and informed decisions about their health and social wellbeing.

In conclusion, providing PSHE can sometimes seem overwhelming because it means tackling potentially sensitive issues. However, it comprises many different activities, which take place across a wide range of settings and periods of time and with lots of opportunities to contribute, not just within a lesson setting. Parents are best placed in relation to young people to provide continuity of individual support and education, and school nurses can support them in this role. School-based education programmes taught by nurses are particularly good at providing factual information and opportunities for skill development and attitude clarification in more formal ways, through lessons within the curriculum. The future of PSHE education depends on joining up these elements in a coherent way to meet young people's needs in order to address health inequalities, and school nurses link the health, education and social services. As the cost to the NHS increases, health education and promotion are becoming more significant and school nurses have an opportunity to influence the population's health before habits become ingrained.

References

Adamson, P. (2007) *Child Poverty in Perspective: An Overview of Child Well-being in Rich Countries*. UNICEF Innocenti Research Centre, Florence.

Ainsworth, P. (2009) Teaching tips for school nurses: organizing effective group work. *British Journal of School Nursing*, **4**(6), 302.

Bennett, S. and Assefi, N. (2005) School-based teenage pregnancy prevention programs: a systematic review of randomized controlled trials. *Journal of Adolescent Health*, **36**(1), 72–81.

Blair, M., Stewart-Brown, S., Waterson, T. and Crowther, R. (2003) *Child Public Health*, p. 178. Oxford University Press, Oxford.

Brook (2008) *Sexual Health Outreach: Why, What and How*. Brook, London.

Caan, W. (2010) Fair society, healthy lives: timing is everything. *British Medical Journal*, March (340), 495.

Change 4 life: http://change4life.icnetwork.co.uk/.

Chamberlain, T., George, N., Golden, S., Walter, F., and Benton, T. (2010) *Tellus4 National Report*. National Foundation for Educational Research, Slough.

Communication Trust, The (2009) *Speech, Language and Communication Information for Secondary School*. The Communication Trust, London.

DeBell, D. and Jackson, P. (2000) *School Nursing Within the Public Health Agenda: A Strategy for Practice*. McMillian-Scott, London.

Department for Children, Schools and Families (2007) *The Children's Plan*. Stationery Office, London.

Department of Children, Schools and Families (2008) *The PE and Sports Strategy*. Available at: https://www.education.gov.uk/publications/eOrderingDownload/PE_Sport_Strategy_leaflet_2008.pdf (accessed 8 October 2011).

Department of Children, Schools and Families (2010) *Sex and Relationships Education Guidance to Schools (Consultation)*. Available at: http://www.education.gov.uk/consultations/index.cfm?action=conResults&consultationId=1637&external=no&menu=3 (accessed 12 October 2011).

Department for Education (2010) *The Importance of Teaching: The Schools White Paper 2010*. Stationery Office, London.

Department for Education (2011) *Review of the National Curriculum in England: Remit*. Available at: http://www.education.gov.uk/schools/teachingandlearning/curriculum/nationalcurriculum/b0073043/remit-for-review-of-the-national-curriculum-in-england/ (accessed: 30 April 2011).

Department of Education and Employment [DfEE] (2000) *Sex and Relationship Education Guidance*. DfEE Publications, Nottingham.

Department for Education and Skills (2004) *PSHE in Practice*. Stationery Office, London.

Department for Education and Skills (2007) *RUThinking (20 March 2007) Tracking Research, Wave 1 Debrief.* Department for Education and Skills Publications, London.

Department of Health (2001) National Strategy for Sexual Health and HIV. Stationery Office, London.

Department of Health (2004a) *Choosing Health: Making Healthy Choices Easier.* Stationery Office, London.

Department of Health (2004b) *National Framework for Children, Young People and Maternity Services.* DH, London.

Department of Health (2005) *Choosing Better Oral Health: An Oral Health Plan for England.* DH, London.

Department of Health (2006) *Our Health, Our care, Our Say.* DH, London.

Department of Health (2007a) *Valuing People's Oral Health: A Good Practice Guide for Improving the Oral Health of Disabled Children and Adults.* DH, London.

Department of Health (2007b) *Smokefree and Smiling: Helping Dental Patients to Quit Tobacco.* DH, London.

Department of Health/Department of Children Schools and Families (2008a) *The Youth Alcohol Action Plan.* DCSF/DH, London.

Department of Health/Department of Children, Schools and Families (2008b) *Healthy Weight, Healthy Lives: Consumer Insight Summary.* Cross-Government Obesity Unit, London.

Department of Health/Department of Children, Schools and Families (2009a) *Healthy Lives, Brighter futures – the Strategy for Children and Young People's Health.* Department of Health Publications, London.

Department of Health/Department for Children, Schools and Families (2009b) *Healthy Child Programme: From 5–19 Years Old.* Department of Health Publications, London.

Department of Health and the British Association for the Study of Community Dentistry (2009) *Delivering Better Oral Health: An Evidence-based Toolkit for Prevention*, 2nd edn. DH/BASCD, London.

Department of Health/Department for Education and Skills (2004) *Every Child Matters – Change for Children.* Stationery Office, London.

Durex, NAHT, NCPTA, NGA (2010) *Sex and Relationship Education: Views Form Teachers, Parents and Governors.* Available at: http://www.durexhcp.co.uk/downloads/SRE-report.pdf (accessed: 12 September 2011).

Emmerson, L. (2011) Provision of sex and relationships education is still not good enough. *British Journal of School Nursing*, 6(5), 218–19.

Family Planning Association (2007) *Are you ready? Young People's Views of Sex and Relationships.* Family Planning Association, London.

Family Planning Association (2011) *Sex and Relationships Education.* Family Planning

181

Association, London.

Gleeson, C. (2001) Children's access to school health nurses. *Primary Health Care*, **11**(9), 33–6.

Hayward, M. (2011) Debate continues over the need for statutory PSHE curriculum. *British Journal of School Nursing*, **6**(5), 248–51.

Health Development Agency (2002) *National Healthy School Standard – School Nursing*. Health Development Agency, Wetherby.

HMSO (1996) *The Education Act*. HMSO, London. Available at: http://www.legislation. gov.uk/ukpga/1996/56/contents (accessed 29 March 2011).

HMSO (1988) *Local Government Act 1988*. HMSO, London. Available at: http://www. legislation.gov.uk/ukpga/1988/9/pdfs/ukpga_ 19880009_en.pdf (accessed 29 March 2011).

HMSO (2000) *Learning and Skills Act*. HMSO, London. Available at: http://www.legisla-tion.gov.uk/ukpga/2000/21/contents (accessed: 29 March 2011).

HM Government (2010) *Healthy Lives, Healthy People: Our Strategy for Public Health in England*. Stationery Office, London.

Hyde, P., McBride, A., Young, R. and Walshe, K. (2005) *Role Redesign: New Ways of Work-ing in the NHS. Personnel Review*, **34**(6), 697–712. Available at: http://www.emeraldin-sight.co/0048-3486.htm (accessed: 12 December 2008).

Kennedy, I. (2010) *Getting it Right for Children and Young People: Overcoming Cultural Barriers in the NHS so as to Meet Their Needs*. Central Office of Information, London.

Kim, C. and Free, C. (2008) Recent evaluations of the peer-led approach in adolescent sexual health education. *International Family Planning Perspectives*, **34**(2), 89–96.

Kochar, R. and Mitchell, L. (2002) *Personal and Social Development, Diversity and Inclu-sion*. NSCoPSE, Doncaster.

Marmot, M. (2010) *Fair Society, Healthy Lives. The Marmot Review*. The Marmot Review, London.

Mages, L., Salmon, D. and Orme, J. (2007) Using drama to help 'hard to reach' young peo-ple access sexual health education. *Primary Health Care*, **17**(4), 41–5.

Morgan, A. and Ziglio, E. (2007) Revitalising the evidence base for public health: an assets model. *Global Health Promotion*, **2** (suppl.), 17–22.

Naidoo, J. and Wills, J. (2005) *Public Health and Health Promotion – Developing Practice* 2nd edn. Baillière Tindall, London.

National Institute of Clinical Excellence (2005) *Health Needs Assessment*. NICE, London.

National Institute for Health and Clinical Excellence (2010) *Public Health Draft Guidance: School, College and Community-based Personal, Social, Health and Economic Educa-tion Focusing on Sex and Relationships and Alcohol Education*. NICE, London.

NSPCC (2009) *NSPCC response to Curriculum Reform Consultation*. NSPCC, London.

Nursing and Midwifery Council (2008) *The Code: Standards of Conduct, Performance and Ethics for Nurses and Midwives*. NMC, London.

Nutbeam, D. (2000) Health literacy as a public health goal: a challenge for contemporary health education and communication strategies into the 21st century. *Health Promotion International*, **15**(3), 259–67.

Office for Standards in Education (2007) *Time for change? Personal, Social and Health Education*. Ofsted, London.

Office for Standards in Education (2010) *Personal, Social, Health and Economic Education in Schools*. Ofsted, London.

PSHE Association (2010) *PSHE Assessing for Learning*. Available at: http://www.pshe-association.org.uk/uploads/media/27/7429.pdf (accessed 30 June 2011).

PSHE Association (2011) *A Briefing for School Governors: Knowing and Understanding Personal, Social, Health and Economic (PSHE) Education in My School*. PSHE Association, London.

Qualifications and Curriculum Authority [QCA] (1999) *The National Curriculum Handbook for Primary Teachers in England Key Stages 1 and 2*. Department for Education and Employment, London.

Qualifications and Curriculum Authority (2007) *The Secondary Curriculum Key Stage 3 and Key Stage 4*. Available at: http://curriculum.qcda. gov.uk/key-stages-3-and-4/ (accessed 30 March 2011).

Royal College of Nursing (2008) *An RCN Toolkit for School Nurses: Developing Your Practice to Support Children and Young People in Educational Settings*. Royal College of Nursing, London.

Sex Education Forum (2000) *Meeting the Needs of Girls and Young Women*. National Children's Bureau for the Sex Education Forum, London.

Sex Education Forum (2002) *Sex and Relationships Education for Primary Age Children*. National Children's Bureau for the Sex Education Forum, London.

Sex Education Forum (2004) *Faith, values and sex and relationships education*. London: National Children's Bureau for the Sex Education Forum

Sex Education Forum (2005a) *Effective Learning Methods*. London: National Children's Bureau for the Sex Education Forum.

Sex Education Forum (2005b) *Sexual orientation, sexual identities and homophobia in schools*. London: National Children's Bureau for the Sex Education Forum.

Sex Education Forum (2006) *Boys and young men: developing effective sex and relationships education in schools*. London: National Children's Bureau for the Sex Education Forum

Sex Education Forum (2008) *Key findings: young people's people's survey on sex and relationships education*. London: National Children's Bureau for the Sex Education Forum.

Sex Education Forum (2011a) *CURRENT status of Sex and Relationships Education*. London: National Children's Bureau for the Sex Education Forum.

Sherbert Research (2009) *Customer Voice Research Sex and Relationship Education*. Department for Children, Schools and Families, London. Available at: https://www.education.gov.uk/publications/eOrdering Download/DCSF-RR175.pdf (accessed 12 October 2011).

Social Exclusion Unit (1999) *Teenage Pregnancy*. HMSO, London.

Standing Nursing and Midwifery Advisory Committee (SNMAC) (2002) *Balancing the Shift – A Position Paper Exploring the Key Issues for Nursing Skill Mix Within the Context of Workforce Planning*. Available at: http://www.dh.gov.uk/en/publicationsandstatistics/publicationspolicyandguidance/DH-4120773 (accessed 16 November 2010).

St Leger, L. (2000) Reducing the barriers to the expansion of health promoting schools by focusing on teachers. *Health Education*, **100**(2), 81–7.

Staffordshire County Council (2008) *Inclusion Development Programme Autism Spectrum*. Available at: http://education.staffordshire.gov.uk/NR/rdonlyres/FD517022-D9E6-4654-90FF-12A16310240E/160759/IDPDyslexiaASstrand.pdf (accessed 22 November 2011).

Stevens, A. and Gilliam, S. (1998) Needs assessment from theory to practice. *British Medical Journal*, **316**, 1448–52.

Tomey, A. (2004) *Guide to Nursing Management and Leadership*, 7th edn. Mosby, Missouri.

Training and Development Agency for Schools. (2009) *Including Pupils with SEN and/or Disabilities in Primary PSHE and Citizenship*. Training and Development Agency for Schools, Manchester.

Underhill, K. (2007) Sexual abstinence only programmes to prevent HIV infection in high income countries: systematic review. *British Medical Journal*, **335**, 248.

UK Youth Parliament (2007) *Are You Getting It?* UK Youth Parliament, London.

Walker, J. L. (2001) A qualitative study of parents' experiences of providing sex education for their children: the implications for health education. *Health Education Journal*, **60**(2), 132–46.

Wanless, D. (2004) *Securing Good Health for the Whole Population. Final Report*. HMSO, London.

Westwood, J. and Mullan, B. (2006) Knowledge of school nurses in the UK regarding sexual health education. *Journal of School Nursing*, **22**(6), 352–7.

Wetton, N. and Williams, T. (2000) *Health for Life – Ages 4–7*. Nelson Thornes, Cheltenham.

Why let drink decide?: http://www.direct.gov.uk/en/Parents/Yourchildshealthandsafety/Youngpeopleandalcohol/index.htm.

CHAPTER 6

Setting up and running a health drop-in

Jane Wright and Rachel Cabral

Key themes in this chapter:

- What are the aims of a health drop-in?
- A step-by-step guide to setting up a drop-in service.
- Confidentiality and Fraser guidelines.
- Responding to need.

> ...The role of the SCPHN is to promote health and a drop-in is an ideal venue to do precisely this. With some imagination, there are no limits to the amount of good a drop-in can do. Imagine running information sessions about 'hot topics' with local young people, inviting in key public figures or services to talk about their area of expertise while allowing young people a place where they know that they can talk to someone about anything and gain some support in their time of need... (Rachel Cabral, School Nurse, 2011)

Introduction

This chapter will explain the complexities of setting up and running a face-to-face health drop-in (HDI) for children and young people in the community setting. There is a place within the school health service for using technology to give advice and provide information, but this chapter will focus on the face-to-face services that remain a valuable resource for many young people. There are a variety of models used across the country, including those that utilise many agencies as well as those run by school nurses alone. There are also other agencies, such as Brook, that run sexual health clinics in schools in different parts of the country. The basic principles of a HDI are that it should provide accessible, confidential services for children and young people. This differs from a referral system that schools may have when they have specific concerns about children and young people, because this is driven by the teachers or educationalists rather than by young people. There is of course, a place for direct referrals, but a HDI service implies that the motivation to attend comes from individuals. Teachers and others may signpost young people to the service, but the ultimate decision about attendance comes young people themselves. This is an 'enabling' or 'empowerment' model of health promotion which has proved to be more effective in establishing sustainable behaviour changes (Farrelly, 2008). It gives control to young people and shows respect for their ability to make decisions about their own health (DH, 2011). A HDI can be set up in both the primary school and secondary school sectors, and consideration should also be given to services in colleges or universities, as the Healthy Child Programme goes up to the 20th birthday (DH/DCSF, 2009). In some areas of the country, school nurses are involved in regular visits to universities to provide sexual health advice and support. However, with limited resources, this could be a neglected area for young people and when they first leave home they may be particularly vulnerable. It is an area for consideration for school health teams across the country.

The driving force for providing these services is to address public health problems such as the rise in teenage pregnancy, an increasing incidence of sexually transmitted infections (STIs), increasing alcohol misuse, and a rise in mental health problems in young people (DH, 2011). However, there are other aspects of a young person's health and wellbeing which are equally important, for example bullying, friendships issues, weight problems, problems related to puberty such as skin complaints and acne, self-esteem issues, poor self-worth, substance misuse, smoking, academic pressures, loss, bereavement, divorce and separation. Understanding a young person's point of view is vital to understanding that what adults may view as 'trivial' is hugely important to the lives of young people. These areas of concern for young people are not always measurable.

The Department of Health document *You're Welcome – Quality Criteria for Young People Friendly Health Services* (DH, 2011) sets out clear guidelines for setting up user-friendly services and forms the basis of this chapter, along with the recommendations from the Health Child Programme (HCP) (DH/DCSF, 2009). A HDI utilises many of the skills and much of the knowledge that a qualified school nurse has and may be considered an important part of the role. Commissioners will need evidence that HDIs are a valuable way of delivering the HCP in order for them to buy those services. Therefore the setting up, running and auditing of these services need to be clearly defined and articulated to commissioners. Essentially, commissioners of services are looking for cost-effective deliverable services that provide value for money (see Chapter 7). The HDI may also form part of a local quality framework (see Box 2.1).

What are the aims of a HDI?

The general aims of a primary school HDI are:

1. To support parents and families in making healthy choices in relation to children and young people.
2. To provide access to health advice and services that may not be otherwise available.
3. To develop trust between health services and vulnerable groups.
4. To contribute to improving the health and wellbeing of the local community.
5. To help build community participation and capacity in maintaining health and wellbeing.
6. To work in partnerships with education and other agencies.
7. To contribute to tackling inequalities.

Some specific issues seen in primary school HDIs are:

- Bullying
- Poor transition into school
- Behavioural problems
- Weight management issues
- Head lice
- Infectious childhood diseases
- Immunisation advice and updates

The general aims of a secondary school HDI service are:

1. To listen to young people and respond to identified needs.
2. To improve young people's access to confidential health services.
3. To promote healthy lifestyles and raise awareness of health-related issues.
4. To encourage and support young people in making informed choices about their health and overall wellbeing.
5. To signpost young people to other services relevant to their health needs.
6. To work collaboratively across relevant agencies.
7. To improve young people's sexual health and help them make sensible choices. This may include chlamydia screening, as recommended in *You're Welcome* (DH, 2011).

Some specific issues seen in secondary school HDIs:

- General physical health issues (for example acne)
- Weight management/nutritional advice/eating disorders, including obesity, bulimia and anorexia
- Free condom distribution (e.g. the 'C Card' Scheme)
- Pregnancy testing
- Signposting to other agencies
- Sexual health advice and screening for STIs (e.g. chlamydia)
- Emotional health and wellbeing support
- Mental health problems
- Self-harming/injuring behaviour
- Smoking
- Substance misuse

The locations of HDIs vary. Some are on school premises and others are off-site in GP practices, health centres or local youth and community premises. Wherever the setting is, a HDI needs to be:

- A comfortable, private place where young people feel safe.
- Easily accessible.
- Open at appropriate times to suit those who are accessing the service, not those who are delivering it.
- A supportive, non-judgemental environment with clear boundaries around child protection.
- Staffed by professional, approachable, friendly staff.

A step-by-step guide to setting up a drop-in service

1. The proposal to provide drop-in services will form part of the commissioned services agreed locally and should involve an integrated team approach. Gain the support of your managers and broader school health team and follow any local guidelines or protocols on developing services. These services should be offered to all schools in the area to ensure parity.
2. Establish the need, listen to the local community. The Healthy Child Programme (DH/DCSF, 2009) recommends robust needs assessments to justify appropriate resources. School nurses may suspect a need through their experiences in the community or in individual schools, but this needs clear evidence to present to service planners (see Chapter 7). One example of clear evidence is in the HCP, which suggests that improving sexual health services could save £500 million over 15 years (DH/DCSF, 2009). This kind

of mathematical modelling and predicting may help to justify services (see Chapter 7).

3. Allow time to establish: don't rush the process. To set up a sustainable HDI means having a sensible lead-in time, which could be up to 18 months to two years.

    Find out as much as you can, network as much as possible, get invited to events or turn up and introduce yourself. Use this time to form an overall picture with which to build your vision for the service you wish to provide. Although it is tempting to want to just push on ahead and get the show up and running, the secret to its true success lies in the ground work. You may find it surprising how much support you will rally along the way, you will also gain some insight into the resistance you may encounter. It would be foolish to pretend that drop-ins are easy to establish, just because we can clearly see the needs and benefits, others often do not. (Rachel Cabral, School Nurse, 2011)

4. Talk to the school staff, head teacher and governors of relevant schools. If the HDI is in school or in school time, you will need to ensure that all these people are engaged in the process from the start. Meet the school governors at one of their meetings to ensure that they are kept fully informed throughout the process.

5. Set up a committee of relevant people and meet regularly to monitor progress and maintain momentum. Find out what is already available to young people in the area and contact them and invite them to join the group. It may be that these services could be utilised either as satellite services in the school or liaison could be improved. You will also need to know this information if you need to signpost young people to their service. Make sure that notes are taken of the meeting to keep everyone motivated and on track. You will get a feel for the commitment of people by holding these meetings regularly.

6. Involve young people in the process; ask them directly what they want. A questionnaire to all pupils is a valuable piece of evidence, and an example template is given in Table 6.1. If possible, let young people name the HDI and suggest a place and time. This gives them ownership and saves you calling the service something which means nothing to them or setting it up where they are unlikely to visit. In some areas, the drop-ins are part of a broader agenda and therefore already named (for example health zones or body zones). Consultation will give you an idea of who they would feel comfortable

Table 6.1 An example questionnaire to pupils

It has been suggested that a health drop-in could be provided at _____ school, where young people could access confidential information, advice and support on a wide range of health issues. Please give us your views by ticking the appropriate boxes. **This is an anonymous questionnaire, so do not put your name on the paper.**

1. **Male** ❑   **Female** ❑

2. **Year Group:**   7   8   9   10   11   12   13   **(please circle)**

3. **Do you think a health drop-in is a good idea?**   Yes ❑   No ❑

4. **What information/advice would you want to find at a health drop-in? (tick all that apply)**

   Diet/eating disorders ❑   Stress/anxiety ❑
   Drugs ❑   Friendship/relationships problems ❑
   Alcohol ❑   Sexual health ❑
   Smoking ❑   Family issues ❑
   Abuse (physical/emotional) ❑   Self-harm ❑
   Bullying ❑   Anger ❑
   General health ❑   Other – please specify:

5. **What professionals would you like to talk to?**
   Doctor/GP ❑   School nurse ❑   Counsellor ❑
   Youth worker ❑   Dietitian ❑   Drug worker ❑
   Other – please specify:

6. **What resources would you like to take away with you?**
   Leaflets ❑   Eating plans ❑   Helpline numbers ❑
   Contraceptive information ❑   Strategies to cope with problems ❑
   Other:

7. **Please tick the most suitable day**
   Monday ❑   Tuesday ❑   Wednesday ❑   Thursday ❑   Friday ❑

8. **Would lunchtime be a suitable time?**
   Yes ❑   No ❑   If No please suggest alternative:

9. **Would you use such a health drop-in if you had a problem?**
   Yes ❑   No ❑   Maybe ❑
   If No please say why:

10. **What would you suggest the health drop-in is called?**

Thank you.

talking to and what kind of advice might be needed. This process also raises awareness of the HDI.

> In these early stages, as well as talking to other professional bodies it is imperative to gauge the thoughts and opinions of those whom you would like to use your service. This can take some effort. Be inventive, if you are running a PSHE session ask them, if you are participating in a school event, ask them, if you are in the school then mill around at break time and ask them (with schools permission). Promote yourself and get their ideas. If the young people don't want the service, will they use it? What would they like from the service if it was available? Start gathering your evidence; you are going to need it when you meet the Governors. (Rachel Cabral, School Nurse, 2011)

7. HDI services need to be agreed by local children's service planners as part of local agreements and there are recommendations in the HCP about improving access to services for young people. Therefore ensure that there is support through the local public health department.

> It is not easy to know when, if or where you might meet resistance along the journey of setting up a drop-in but if you do, it is helpful to be prepared. Having done your background research and gathered your evidence, presenting the evidence could 'make or break' the project. It may be becoming clear now that as a school nurse not only do you need all the skills you spent an intense year training for, you also need detective skills, market research skills, networking skill, and, be the salesperson, deciding how to sell your 'pitch'. (Rachel Cabral, School Nurse, 2011)

8. Use local policy guidelines on setting up a drop-in. If these are not in place, ensure that they are developed with all the relevant stakeholders and that the service is considering broader relevant public health agendas (for example obesity or sexual health). There are good examples of protocols which are in the public domain and can be accessed online. It is important to coordinate these protocols across a Trust to ensure parity across the schools – this reduces inequality. The *You're Welcome* (DH, 2011) guidance should be followed, and this is available at:

> http://www.dh.gov.uk/en/Publicationsandstatistics/
> Publications/PublicationsPolicyAndGuidance/DH_126813

It includes a self-assessment tool which covers the following themes:

- Universal services:
  - Accessibility
  - Publicity
  - Confidentiality and consent
  - Environment
  - Staff training, skills, attitudes, values
  - Joined-up working
  - Involvement of young people in feedback, monitoring and evaluation
  - Health issues for adolescents

There are two further themes focusing on specialist and targeted provision:

- Sexual and reproductive health services
- Specialist and targeted child and adolescent mental health services (CAMHS)

This guidance can be used to develop the protocols.

Other key areas to consider in a HDI framework/protocol are:

- Clarity of purpose: what exactly will the HDI deliver?
- Duration of project and auditing procedures.
- Confidentiality.
- Safeguarding and child protection.
- Professional accountability.
- Clear protocols in the provision of contraceptives or pregnancy testing. Consider guidelines for young people under 13 years old.
- Use of Patient Group Directives for any medications, for example contraceptives.

9. It is a good idea to use this opportunity to link in with a school's PSHE curriculum. Becoming part of the delivery of the sex and relationships education (SRE) will enable you to advertise the drop-in and begin to establish trusting relationships with young people. See Chapter 5 for more details on SRE.

10. Staff training is essential. Qualified school nurses have the knowledge and skills to understand the needs of young people and be able to communicate effectively. All those working in the HDI will need to be following clear guidelines, and lines of accountability and responsibilities should be established from the start. The key knowledge and skills for all those working with children and young people are outlined in *The Common Core of Skills and Knowledge for the Children's Workforce* (HM Government, 2005):

- Effective communication and engagement with children, young people, their families and carers.
- Understanding of child development.
- Understanding the duty of care to safeguard and promote the welfare of children and young people.
- Support transitions.
- Work together and share information in order to act in the best interests of children and young people.

11. You will need to evaluate the service. This means recording the numbers visiting the service, the reasons for the visits and the ages and gender of the young people. This will enable you to monitor and change the service according to need and remarket the service if necessary. The NHS Information Centre (2011) and the Centre for Excellence and Outcomes for children and young people (C4EO, 2011) gather information and publish data related to children and young people. C4EO can provide support for projects and advice on auditing services, but it is also an organisation that publishes examples of good practice (C4EO, 2011). The key issue is that a service should provide 'value for money' and the Audit Commission (2009) provides a good definition of this: 'making the best use of available resources, including getting better outcomes for the same spend, or freeing up resources that are being used inefficiently for other purposes'. For example, qualified school nurses can be 'freed' up to run HDIs if they utilise skill mix and use other staff appropriately (see Chapter 7). Local areas will have quality governance departments and their role is to measure the effectiveness of services and set standards for care. You will need to work closely with them to monitor the outcomes of the service and set quality benchmarks.

Building partnerships: who do you need to build partnerships with?

- Young people
- Head teachers
- Teachers and pastoral care leads in schools
- Governors
- Parents
- Local public health/health promotion departments
- Health services such as GPs, sexual health services and pharmacists
- Mental health services
- Youth services
- Drugs and alcohol teams

School nurses require good communication and negotiating skills to justify the service to key stakeholders and commissioners (see Chapter 2).

It may be you need to meet with the school and the governors on more than one occasion, initially present the idea and give them time to discuss it and return a few weeks later to respond to questions and re-visit the topic. People need time to think about the issues that may be worrying them. No matter who you talk to, how exciting a package you present to those in authority, the true test of whether this venture will be successful is how 'users' have been engaged in the process. It can be challenging to get their input and involvement over a prolonged period of time but they can be powerful champions with a wealth of ideas and motivated and enthusiastic volunteers can be instrumental in the success of the drop-in.' (Rachel Cabral, School Nurse, 2011)

It is essential that school nurses create a contact list of other agencies who work with young people in the local area and gather information about their services and what they offer. This can be achieved by networking in a number of ways:

- Attending local conferences
- Study days
- Updates and training days
- Local data through health and local authority services
- GP surgeries
- Websites

With limited resources and staffing and funding issues, gaining a regular commitment from a partner agency may be problematic, but it is essential for sustainability. Utilising limited resources to best effect is crucial to success (see Chapter 7).

What other agencies could I be working with?
- Local drugs and alcohol services, such as addictions specialist workers
- Homeless persons outreach workers
- CAMHS workers
- Youth services
- GPs
- Sexual health staff

Training staff

There will be universal training, that all staff will need to attend, which addresses health and safety in the workplace as well as risk management. This will include regular, multi-agency child protection training. The purpose of a drop-in is to offer young people a place where they feel safe to talk, so it is likely that a child protection issue will arise at some point (see Chapter 4). Understanding of current child protection guidelines, both national and local, is therefore essential (see Chapter 4).

Training will also be needed to provide good sexual health services. If a condom distribution service has been agreed, then young people need to be given accurate information and a demonstration of how to use them effectively. Operating in many areas is the C-Card scheme. This is a free and confidential scheme, providing condoms, advice and information targeted at young people. The aim is to enable young people to get condoms more easily and without embarrassment. There is an initial consultation with a trained sexual health advisor where the young person is given information about correct usage, what to do if a condom breaks and who to contact if there are any concerns. This initial consultation also allows the health professional to assess any other health needs, as well as the level of maturity of the young person, and advise accordingly. The young person is given a card which they can use at a number of outlets which have signed up to the scheme. They can then access new supplies without further consultation and the card is usually valid for a set number of visits and 'stamped' at each visit. This is useful because, once the card is 'full' the young person needs another consultation. This will allow health professionals to reassess their individual health needs. Regular training and updating on this is important to ensure that correct information is given to young people regarding sexual health.

Equally, with pregnancy testing, careful questioning and a thorough assessment are important. A sensitive approach is clearly needed with young people to establish their understanding of sexual health, sexuality and risk-taking behaviour. Sexual health forms a key part of the Healthy Child Programme (HCP), given the rise in STIs and the level of teenage pregnancy, and, therefore, sexual health services are a recommended at a local level (DH/DCSF, 2009). Some schools may be reluctant to include sexual health in the HDI, but evidence suggests that young people may ask about sexual health in a drop-in even if they are accessing the service for other reasons. Knowledge of other services to refer young people on to is key if the school is reluctant to offer these services. Once the HDI is running, a record of the enquiries around sexual health will be important evidence for schools to provide these services if the need is there.

Confidentiality

One of the primary concerns for young people about accessing health services is around confidentiality (DH, 2011). While complete confidentiality should never be promised to young people, they need to be confident that you will act in their best interests and you must be clear from the outset about this. A statement of confidentiality should be agreed as part of the protocols set up for the drop-in and should include information that if there are concerns about someone's safety, this may be shared with appropriate people. An example of a confidentiality statement is in Box 6.1.

Box 6.1 An example confidentiality statement

All staff working in sexual health services have to keep any information about you confidential. They are there to listen, not to tell.

Sexual health is very personal and any questions asked are only to make sure that you receive the right tests and the right care.

If you are under 16 you have the same right of confidentiality as an adult. However, by law you are asked some extra questions to make sure you understand what will happen to you when attending the clinic.

Staff are not allowed to share information outside of the staff in this service unless there is a medical need or because someone's safety is at risk (and then only if they are involved with your care). Laws safeguarding under 16s can occasionally overrule the absolute confidentiality of the clinic. It is very rare that this needs to happen and it would always be discussed with you first. It would only ever be necessary to protect you from harm.

The law on consent and confidentiality

In 1982, Victoria Gillick famously took West Norfolk and Wisbech Area Health Authority and the Department for Health and Social Security (DHSS) to court for providing a minor (her daughter) with contraceptive treatment without parental knowledge. The DHSS had issued guidance in 1980 for family planning services which said that in exceptional circumstances, a doctor (or other professional) could give contraceptive advice and treatment to girls under 16. Mrs Gillick claimed that this guidance was unlawful. The courts ruled in her favour, basing their decision on existing laws about unlawful sex with girls under 16, 'incitement' by a doctor to have unlawful sex and parental responsibility. The Department of Health and Social Security then appealed the decision in the High Court, where the appeal was upheld and the original decision set aside. Lord Fraser of Tullybelton, Lord Scarman, Lord Bridge of Harwich, Lord Brandon of Oakbrook and Lord Templeman were the Lords who gave statements in this case (Gillick, 1985). The statements were not all in favour of setting aside the original decision, but Lord Fraser and Lord Scarman gave particularly compelling arguments. This ruling has formed the basis of the guidelines for sexual health services for young people and they have become known as the Fraser guidelines (or ruling). Lord Fraser clarified that he was not just referring to doctors in the decision:

> ...I shall refer throughout to doctors, to include *bevitatis causa* other professional persons working in the NHS... (Gillick, 1985, p. 5)

This is an important clarification for school nurses and others working in HDIs that provide sexual health services.

The key issues in providing sexual health and advice centre around:

- the capacity of young people under 16 to 'understand';
- their competency to consent;
- their rights; and
- parents' rights.

Lord Fraser agreed that professionals could provide advice and treatment to young people under 16:

> ...Provided the patient, whether a boy or a girl, is capable of understanding what is proposed, and of expressing his or her own wishes, I see no good reason for holding that he or she lacks the capacity to express them validly and effectively and to authorise the medical man [professional] to make the examination or give the treatment which he advises.... I conclude that there is no statutory provision which compels me to hold that a girl under the age of 16 lacks the legal capacity to consent to contraceptive advice, examination and treatment provided that she has sufficient understanding and intelligence to know what they involve... (Gillick, 1985, pp. 6 and 7)

The issue around this capability to understand or competency to consent is a contentious one and was debated by the Lords in the Gillick case. How is the ability to 'understand' judged for example? This rests with the professional on a case by case basis, and in making decisions they should be confident that they can justify their choice; clearly, this takes training and experience. School nurses are experienced in talking to young people on a regular basis and one could argue that they are in a strong position to make these judgements about a level of understanding. Child protection training should also underpin this with regard to acting in the best interests of the child or young person.

The professional must establish that all of the following criteria are met (Gillick, 1985):

- *The young person will understand the advice and the moral, social and emotional implications.*

  Establishing that the sexual relationship is not an abusive one will be important for school nurses. How old is the partner for example? Sex with a girl aged between 13 and 16 is an offence; however, the law will take the age difference between young people into account. Does the young person also understand what sexual intercourse actually is and what the risks are? The myths that still exist around sex need to be dispelled at this point. There have been examples of sex and relationship education being delivered by people who lack knowledge themselves and have perpetuated some of these myths to young people. A good example of this is that you 'cannot get pregnant if you have sex during a period'. Clearly, inaccurate information that needs to be explained when young people access sexual health services.

- *The young person cannot be persuaded to tell their parents or allow the [doctor] to tell them that they are seeking contraceptive advice.*

  There is recognition in a majority of cases that parents are the best people to give advice and support for their children with regard to sexual health (see Chapter 5). However, school nurses recognise that young people can find it difficult to approach this topic with their parents. Parents can also be reluctant to talk about sex – it makes them feel uncomfortable and they can have difficulty acknowledging that their children may want to have sex. In addition to HDIs, advice to parents generally about how to talk to their children is good practice and school nurses are in a good position to do this (see Chapter 5).

- *The young person is having, or is likely to have, unprotected sex whether they receive advice or not.*

  School nurses, through good communication will be able to ascertain this information.

- *Their physical or mental health is likely to suffer unless they receive the advice or treatment.*

  The risks of teenage pregnancy or contracting sexually transmitted infections has the potential to impact on a young person's physical and mental health in the long term and this needs to be considered and discussed with the young person.

■ *It is in the young person's best interest to give contraceptive advice or treatment without parental consent.*
Guidance in the NMC code (NMC, 2008) endorses this. Disclosing information to parents may put young people at further risk, and this needs to be judged on a case by case basis.

Young people's rights and parental rights

As well as discussion around the capacity to understand in order to give consent, some of the debate in the Gillick case was around balancing the rights of young people against parental rights. Laws dating back to the Victorian era were explored where parents, particularly fathers, had the right to 'control' their children. Lord Fraser and Lord Scarman discussed this in relation to the changes that occur in society and they made some interesting points in relation to sexual health services. Lord Scarman argued that:

> ...Three features have emerged in today's society which were not known to our predecessors:- (1) contraception as a subject for medical advice and treatment; (2) the increasing independence of young people; and (3) the changed status of women. In times past contraception was rarely a matter for the doctor: but with the development of the contraceptive pill for women it has become part and parcel of every-day medical practice... (Gillick, 1985, p. 21)

Lord Fraser also highlighted a sensible view of parents' rights:

> ...that parental rights to control a child do not exist for the benefit of the parent. They exist for the benefit of the child and they are justified only in so far as they enable the parent to perform his duties towards the child, and towards other children in the family... (Gillick, 1985, p. 9)

Parenting capacity is often discussed when there are concerns about children and young people and the skills of parents to 'manage' their children are often criticised for not maintaining enough control. There have been calls for parents to be held more responsible for their children's behaviour, for example ensuring that their children attend school or when children are 'anti-social'. What is clear is that the development of children through adolescence into adulthood can be a traumatic one for both parents and young people, and the school nurse role is to support them through this transition. The key to the transition is developing independence, and Lord Fraser argued that:

...In practice most wise parents relax their control gradually as the child develops and encourages him or her to become increasingly independent. Moreover, the degree of parental control actually exercised over a particular child does in practice vary considerably according to his understanding and intelligence and it would, in my opinion, be unrealistic for the courts not to recognise these facts... (Gillick, 1985, p. 10)

The 'just say no' argument

Against the flow of the arguments put forward by Lord Fraser and Lord Scarman in particular during the Gillick case, Lord Brandon of Oakbrook suggested that:

...if all a girl under 16 needs to do in order to obtain contraceptive treatment is to threaten that she will go ahead with, or continue, unlawful sexual intercourse with a man unless she is given such treatment, a situation tantamount to blackmail will arise which no legal system ought to tolerate. The only answer which the law should give to such a threat is 'wait till you are 16'.

The ideas around abstaining from sex have been emerging in the UK in recent years and originate in the USA (see Chapter 5). Nadine Dorries, Conservative MP for Mid Bedfordshire, put forward a private member's bill in 2011 calling for girls to be given mandatory abstinence lessons. It was withdrawn in January 2012 before being debated in the House of Commons. This may be reflective of the lack of real evidence that teaching abstinence in schools affects the rates of teenage pregnancy or the rate of sexually transmitted infections (see Chapter 5). There was also visible objection to this bill, with parents demonstrating outside the House of Commons.

Young people below the age of 13

There is a general consensus that young people below the age of 13 will rarely have the capacity or competence to be able to consent without parental involvement. However, this remains debatable given cases of young people under 13 being involved in violent crime and the question of culpability that these raise, or those instances of young people under 13 becoming parents. An assessment of competence should be made on an individual basis, but it can be a difficult dilemma for school nurses. Clear guidelines should be written into the protocols. The following Family Planning Association guidelines may be helpful when talking to young people under 16:

The Sexual Offences Act 2003 introduced a new series of laws to protect children under 16 from sexual abuse. However, the law is not intended to prosecute mutually agreed teenage sexual activity between two young people of a similar age, unless it involves abuse or exploitation (FPA, 2011).

Specific laws protect children under 13, who cannot legally give their consent to any form of sexual activity. There is a maximum sentence of life imprisonment for rape, assault by penetration, and causing or inciting a child to engage in sexual activity. There is no defence of mistaken belief about the age of the child, as there is in cases involving 13–15 year olds (FPA, 2011).

Conclusion

If you really want to know how young people think and how they are living their lives, then work at a drop-in. Young people have a huge capacity to allow us insight into how they 'tick' and are often unfairly represented in the media today. The most valuable source of information about what young people need comes directly from them. Take time to listen, challenge their ideas, ask them the questions, what, why, where, when how? Then take all this information in and ask them, what would they like? If they are all smoking, would they like to give up? You could pull in support and create a stop smoking group. Are they all drinking? Let's get alcohol workers in to talk about safe drinking. The beauty of the drop-in is you can address issues as they arise and it allows you to plan for the younger groups. Does the school have a common theme of cyber bullying or bereavement? Maybe there are groups of youngsters engaging in risky behaviours. Collating information does not mean identifying individuals or groups but it allow us to plan and bring in the right services to the area. Each school will have a pressing issue; none will necessarily be at the same time. (Rachel Cabral, School Nurse, 2011)

Health drop-ins have the potential to be responsive to the needs of young people locally. Keeping records of attendance and what issues are commonly presented will be important evidence for commissioners. Outcomes are also crucial, so recording the results of interventions will also be important to justify services. Direct links can be made between a drop-in and the PSHE in the school, and where school nurses are not involved in the PSHE delivery the drop-in may provide evidence for them to become involved (see Chapter 5).

General helplines and links

British Pregnancy Advisory Service: http://www.bpas.org/bpaswoman; Tel: 0845 730 4030

NHS Sexual Health Helpline: Tel: 0800 567123

Brook: http://www.brook.org.uk/; Tel: 0800 0185 023

Sexperience: http://sexperienceuk.channel4.com/

Childline – 24 hour free, confidential helpline: http://www.childline.org.uk/; Tel: 0800 1111

MIND (Mental health support): http://www.mind.org.uk/; Tel: 0845 766163

NHS Direct: http://www.nhsdirect.nhs.uk/; Tel: 0845 46 47

Crimestoppers: http://www.crimestoppers-uk.org/; Tel: 0800 555 111

Youth Health Talk: http://www.youthhealthtalk.org/

Sex Worth Talking About – Tel: 0800 282930. Information on sex, relationships and contraception. Will provide details about local services.

Like It Is – Information for teenagers about sex and sexual health: http://www.likeitis.org/

Education for Choice – Information on pregnancy choices, including abortion: http://www.efc.org.uk/

References

Audit Commission (July 2009) *Valuable Lessons: Improving Economy and Efficiency in Schools*. Audit Commission, London.

C4EO (2011) General website available at: http://www.c4eo.org.uk/.

Department of Health/Department for Children, Schools and Families (2009) *Healthy Child Programme: From 5–19 Years Old*. Department of Health Publications, London.

Department of Health (2011) *You're Welcome – Quality Criteria for Young People Friendly Health Services*. DH, London.

Farrelly, P. (2008) Models of health promotion in action: what works? In: *Promoting the Health of School Age Children* (eds. V. Thurtle and J. Wright). Quay Books, London.

FPA (2011) *The Law on Sex Factsheet*. Available at: http://www.fpa.org.uk/professionals/factsheets/lawonsex (accessed 15 January 2012).

Gillick v. West Norfolk and Wisbech Area Health Authority (1985) [Gillick, 1985] UKHL 7 (17 October 1985). Available at the British and Irish Legal Information Institute (BAILII) website: http://www.bailii.org/uk/cases/UKHL/1985/7.html

HM Government (2005) *The Common Core of Skills and Knowledge for the Children's Workforce*. Stationery Office, London.

The NHS Information Centre (2011) General website available at: http://www.ic.nhs.uk/.

CHAPTER 7

Developing school nursing practice

Kath Lancaster

Key themes in this chapter:

- Implementing new ways of working:
    - What is the School Nurse Development Programme?
    - What will it mean to qualified school nurses?
- Understanding commissioning:
    - How do the stages of the commissioning process work?
    - What does the commissioning process mean to school nursing?
    - How to influence the commissioning process
- Essential steps to writing a business plan:
    - What is a business plan?
    - How to write a business plan using a basic template
- Improving the efficiency of teams: the Lancaster Model

Introduction

This chapter will explore the development of school nursing practice in response to changing health and social care agendas, changes to the NHS and the restructuring of public health services. School nurses will have to consider new ways of working which involve thinking more strategically, understanding the commissioning cycle and using resources more effectively and efficiently to address the needs of children and young people in the future. School nurses remain a key point of contact for young people aged 5 to 19 and are leaders in the delivery of the Healthy Child Programme (HCP), as discussed in previous chapters (DH/DCSF, 2009). The school nurse's contribution to this delivery will be explored further in this chapter and the School Nurse Development Programme (SNDP) summarised. There will also be discussion of some of the models and frameworks that support successful delivery of services.

Implementing new ways of working

What is the School Nurse Development Programme?

The School Nurse Development Programme (SNDP) (DH, 2012) was a collaborative directive led by the Department of Health (DH) in 2011 to clarify the valuable contribution that the school nursing service offers and its unique contribution to improving the health and wellbeing of school-aged children and young people (CNO, 2011). The SNDP was designed to support the development of a strengthened and well-equipped school nurse workforce. The overall aim is to enable school nursing teams to increase their public health involvement with school-age children, young people and their families and deliver the *Healthy Child Programme 5–19* (DH/DCSF, 2009). The whole approach aimed to build on *The Action for Health Visiting Programme* (DH, 2010), based on the enhancement of service provision at community, universal, universal plus and universal partnership plus level. A summary of the SNDP model is contained in Box 7.1.

Box 7.1 Overview of the SNDP model

The school nurse development model
The offer

- **Your community** has a range of health services (including GP and community services) for children and young people and their families. School nurses develop and provide these and make sure you know about them
- **Universal services** from your school nurse team provide the Healthy Child Programme to ensure a healthy start for every child (e.g. immunisations, health checks). They support children and parents to ensure access to a range of community services.
- **Universal plus** delivers a swift response from your school nurse service when you need specific expert help (e.g. with sexual health, mental health concerns, long-term conditions and additional health needs).
- **Universal partnership plus** delivers ongoing support by your school nursing team from a range of local services working together and with you, to deal with more complex issues over a period of time (e.g. with charities and your local authority).

What will it mean to qualified school nurses?
The delivery of school nursing services will become more visible, standardised and proactive. Qualified school nurses will be the health leaders for school-aged children, young people and their families within the wider multi-agency team.

There are four principal areas of practice which qualified school nurses will need to focus on:

1. Managing and delivering the Healthy Child Programme
The Healthy Child Programme is a good practice guide outlining recommendations for a universal service to promote optimal health and wellbeing and the additional services for those with specific needs and risk factors (see Chapter 1). Specifically, at key transition points, children and young people's health will need to be reviewed. This means that each individual child at school entry (aged 4–5 years) and each young person in Year 6 (aged 10–11 years) will require a universal contact in the form of a health and development review. These reviews will be monitored and measured to ensure that service offers are equitable and available for all.

Each health and development review will:

- Assess strengths, needs and risks
- Provide the opportunity to discuss concerns and aspirations
- Assess physical health, growth and development
- Assess any mental or emotional issues
- Identify any needs which require progressive (targeted) interventions
- Ensure appropriate support is available

2. Team leadership and delegation
In order to maximise resources within existing teams and achieve the school nurse development model, qualified school nurses will be required to delegate practice and utilise the expertise of all team members. This will involve providing measurable outcomes and ensuring that each task or intervention delegated appropriately matches an individual's skills and competencies. Suitable caseload allocation will help to improve team and partnership working, resulting in the right person with the right skills delivering the right services.

3. Early help, intervention, support and referral
The case for prevention and early intervention is reinforced within the HCP and the School Nurse Development Programme and will therefore certainly direct school nursing services in the future. Qualified school nurses will be required to provide the evidence to identify and support proactive earlier interventions for

children, young people and their families. Referrals to other skilled professionals in the wider multi-agency team will increase as needs and problems are identified and uncovered earlier on a universal level. New pathways and referral systems will develop. However, they may differ at a local level, depending on local need and existing multi-agency team compositions.

4. Developing and delivering public health programmes
The focus of any public health programme is to improve health and quality of life through prevention, surveillance and the promotion of healthy behaviours. The *Healthy Child Programme* and the School Nurse Development Model both focus on prevention, surveillance and the healthy behaviours of children, young people and their families. Qualified school nurses are highly-skilled professionals equipped to lead and deliver effective public health programmes. The leadership, development and delivery of these programmes will become the most prominent part of a qualified school nurse's role. Each public health programme must be based on evidence, focused on population health needs and contribute to children and young people's health and wellbeing.

What will change at practice level?
The four principal areas of practice will initiate direct changes at practice level. These changes will also support the commissioning process with measurable outcomes and evidence for future investment.

1. Leading and delivering the Healthy Child Programme
A structured assessment of need will be required for every single child at school entry (aged 4–5 years) and every young person in Year 6 (aged 10–11 years) regardless. Logistically it would be impossible to provide a face-to-face contact to all children and young people at these two stages; however, a structured process of needs assessment that incorporates health and development reviews will enable existing teams to deliver the Healthy Child Programme and provide the evidence to prioritise and deliver the appropriate targeted services. The means by which this process is delivered will be decided locally, but school nurse leaders should be contributing to these decisions and consider the most efficient and practical way to review children at these stages of development.

2. Team leadership, referral and delegation
The correct use of skill mix will be paramount within school nursing teams; any delegation of interventions to team members must be aligned to their skills and competencies and directed by structured pathways of care to improve team

productivity. To support this, the roles and responsibilities of each team member will need to be specific and within competency and capability levels. All team members will benefit from clear boundaries and role clarity and an understanding of their accountability, responsibility and areas of practice. Transparent practice boundaries will help to increase corporate working and team vision, with all team members understanding and recognising their strengths and limitations. Recognition of qualifications, experience and knowledge, regardless of band level, will help individuals to feel motivated and competent. It is essential that staff caseloads become equitable and balanced and directed by the needs of communities and the skills and competencies of the staff. Effective leadership and appropriate delegation of work from the qualified school nurses will help to maximise resources, increase team productivity and utilise the expertise of all team members (see Chapters 2 and 3).

3.   Early help, intervention, support and referral

Early help, support and referral for children, young people and their families will be the most significant change for school nursing services. This proactive approach will only be achieved by way of the successful implementation of the health and development reviews as recommended in the Healthy Child Programme. The information and data collated via each health and development review will require analysis and scrutiny to ensure that identifying indicators and needs-led evidence can validate and support earlier interventions and practices. This may involve letting go of some present practices and embracing new ones to reflect an increase in proactive prevention rather than reactive maintenance.

4.   Developing and delivering public health programmes

Qualified school nurses will need to take on the public health lead for school-aged children and young people, utilising their public health training into practice and achieving the standards of proficiency. The Nursing and Midwifery Council (NMC) established Part 3 of the nursing register specifically for Specialist Community Public Health Nurses – SCPHN (qualified school nurses), taking the view that this form of practice required distinct standards of proficiency (NMC, 2004). These standards of proficiency underpin the ten key principles of public health practice in the context of specialist public health nursing, and include:

- Searching for health needs
- Working with and for communities
- Providing new innovative services
- Leading and facilitating people and resources to improve health and wellbeing

Developing and delivering public health programmes will become a principal role for all qualified school nurses. This will involve delivering these distinct standards of proficiency and leading and facilitating teams to be more cost effective by preventing ill health rather than treating established disease (see Chapter 1).

What are the steps to ensure effective delivery?
There are four steps that qualified school nurses will need to take to ensure effective delivery of the School Nurse Development Model (DH, 2012). These steps have been aligned to service provision at community, universal, universal plus and universal partnership plus level (Table 7.1).

Understanding commissioning
Primarily, commissioning is a structured way of deciding how and on whom public money should be spent. The structured approach is presented as a step-by-step progression that helps prioritise the resources available for service users. Commissioning exists to secure the best outcomes for communities by making use of all available resources to ensure that needs are met (DH, 2009a)

The principles of commissioning are relatively standard across all organisations and relate to the following areas:

- Involving stakeholders
- Forming relationships
- Understanding needs
- Wider outcomes
- Commissioning together
- Sharing resources
- Managing markets
- Innovation
- Transforming services
- Managing performance
- Evaluation

Commissioners are increasingly becoming advocates for health and wellbeing, encouraging and enabling individuals, families and communities to take greater and shared responsibility for staying healthy and managing their health and conditions. Part of the commissioning role means understanding better the determinants of health, effective engagement and enablement of people and populations to improve health and wellbeing. The discipline of school nursing is in an exclusive position to provide commissioners with a vast source of information and data with

Table 7.1 Four steps to practice.

Step 1 **Scope and** **understand** (the Your Community element)	Qualified school nurse to initiate: ■ Profile your schools and their communities ■ Identify the range of services available in your community ■ Provide data and information to evidence your understanding
Step 2 **Needs assessment** (the Universal Services element)	Qualified school nurse to lead and facilitate: ■ Assess the needs of *all* children at school entry (aged 4–5 years) and Year 6 (aged 10–11 years) ■ Ensure inclusion of health and development reviews ■ Collate and analyse all the needs assessment information ■ Provide robust evidence of the needs based on a structured, measurable approach
Step 3 **Follow up** (the Universal Plus element)	Qualified school nurse to delegate and oversee: ■ Identify individual children and their families with problems who may require further interventions ■ Respond swiftly with either secondary assessment or additional brief interventions ■ Utilise the skills and competencies of team to follow up effectively ■ Identify population public health issues and prioritise accordingly
Step 4 **Collaborative** **working** (the Universal Partnership Plus element)	Qualified school nurse to facilitate: ■ Ensure ongoing support for individual children from within the team ■ Refer others on to the appropriate service or agency via Pathways of Care ■ Share population data with the wider team and appropriate agencies ■ Work together with others to plan and deliver community public health interventions/sessions ■ Monitor and evaluate service delivery

regard to the health and wellbeing of children, young people and their families. The challenge ahead is ensuring that the content, validity, relevance and delivery of this information and data supports and influences the commissioning cycle.

What is the commissioning cycle?

The commissioning cycle is a process to assess the suitability of service provision and delivery within the NHS (DH, 2009b). This repeated approach includes the development, review and approval of three separate plans:

1. The **strategic commissioning plan**, which determines the provider organisation's direction and priorities for at least the next five years.
2. The **operating plan**, which sets out how the provider organisation plans to achieve the health outcomes and financial goals set out in the strategic commissioning plan.
3. The **organisational development plan**, which concentrates on the organisational capabilities and what is needed to deliver the strategic commissioning plan.

The key to the successful development and delivery of the three commissioning plans is the appropriate, timely information and evidence to direct decision making. There are many different models of the commissioning cycle; these various models often look different if presented graphically. However, although the language may differ and the steps may be divided in various ways and with different emphases, the fundamental elements in the process are common.

How do the stages of the commissioning process work?
There are four essential stages required within the commissioning process to substantiate the effective and efficient planning of health provision (Figure 7.1). Each stage represents an element of a reflective progression.

1. Understand
Local need, resources and existing practice will be identified at this stage to define how future service provision will be configured. This stage must include user involvement; it goes beyond just consultation and should mean effective engagement between commissioners, service providers and users.

The understand stage involves:

- Assessing needs
- Mapping supply
- Identifying all resources

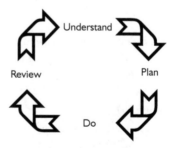

Figure 7.1 The four stages of the commissioning process.

2. Plan

This stage involves defining priorities and agreeing outcomes. Resources must be used creatively to add value and develop services in the right place, at the right time, provided by the right people.

The planning stage involves:

- Setting priorities
- Agreeing desired outcomes
- Designing and planning services
- Developing the commissioning strategy and procurement plan

3. Do

This is the decision-making stage when service specifications are agreed. Mechanisms will be developed to procure both current and new services; however, there is a possibility that some services may be removed from an existing provider.

The 'doing' stage involves:

- Developing and shaping the market
- Securing and decommissioning services

4. Review

This is the monitoring stage, when commissioners will be striving for continuous improvement. Delivery options will be reviewed and measured against the agreed outcomes and staff performance, with an overall goal of value for money.

The reviewing stage involves:

- Monitoring and managing performance
- Evaluating
- Reassessing strategy

What are commissioning and provider indicators?

Commissioning and provider indicators are the measurements used to support the commissioning process. There are a wide variety of indicators currently available. However, all providers of health care are in an extremely strong position to help influence future service provision.

1. Understand

Firstly, it is essential that commissioners understand the needs of children, young people and their families at both an individual and population level (Table 7.2). Further knowledge with regard to the skills and competencies of school nursing teams, users' views and aspirations, current service delivery and any gaps

Table 7.2 Influencing indicators.

Commissioning indicators	Provider indicators
Joint needs assessment (JNSA)	Structured process to identify need
World class commissioning data packs	User involvement information
Public health information	Workforce skills analysis
Workforce statistics	Scoping exercise/benchmark
	Gaps analysis

in provision will enhance their appreciation of the requirements to deliver the appropriate services and interventions.

2. Plan

Based on the information and evidence provided, commissioners next map out and consider the services and interventions required to meet the identified need. Certainly returns on investment (ROI) and school nursing policy will dictate decision making, and therefore will be powerful key indicators (Table 7.3).

Table 7.3 Influencing indicators.

Commissioning indicators	Provider indicators
Payment by results/costs	Local priorities
Hospital admissions	Returns on investment
The Secondary Users Service (SUS)	Policy directives
	Risk assessment

3. Do

Commissioners will work in partnership with providers and potential providers to ensure diversity of supply, choice, contestability, quality and sustainability. During this stage school nursing teams can take the opportunity to provide the evidence to support value for money. New ways of working will be considered at this stage in the process, and some services may be decommissioned if unsuccessful or expensive, or outcomes cannot be measured (Table 7.4).

Table 7.4 Influencing indicators.

Commissioning indicators	Provider indicators
Workforce planning	Monitor and evaluate existing
World class commissioning data packs	interventions
Value for money	Prove outcomes
	Show effectiveness, efficiency and productivity
	New ways of working

4. Review

Ongoing data relating to practice activity and the changing needs of specific users will be required to ensure service delivery is monitored against expected outcomes. During this stage, it is crucial for school nursing teams to continually evaluate their practice, demonstrate specific outcomes and show improvements in effectiveness and productivity (Table 7.5).

Table 7.5 Influencing indicators.

Commissioning indicators	Provider indicators
Quality and outcomes framework (QOF)	Robust service evaluation
Patient records outcome measures	Staff performance data
(PROMS)	Practice activity measurements
Indicators for quality improvements (IQI)	Ongoing needs assessment data

What does commissioning mean to school nursing teams?

Appropriate information and evidence are the key to the successful development and delivery of the three commissioning plans. School nursing teams must provide adequate information and suitable evidence to feed in to strategic planning and show the uniqueness and necessity of their role. Insufficient data may result in reduced investment and ultimately a reduction in service provision for children, young people and their families. Commissioning provides an opportunity and structure to support the future development of school nursing, increased understanding and positive recognition of this from all team members, will ultimately result in more strategic investment and a happier workforce.

Essential steps to writing a business plan

What is a business plan?

A business plan is a formal statement of a set of goals, the reasons why they are believed attainable, and the plan for reaching those goals. A business plan helps allocate resources, focus on key points, and prepare for problems and opportunities (New Economics Foundation, 2009). Unfortunately, many people think this formal approach is only for either starting up a new business or applying for business loans. However, this is an essential method of data presentation which school nursing teams can adopt to influence the four stages of the commissioning process.

Why write a business plan?

Once the appropriate information and evidence has been collated by school nursing teams, this should be presented to commissioners in a comprehensive, readable format.

Firstly, answer the following three leading questions:

1. **What are you actually aiming to achieve and how are you going to achieve it?**

   Can you:
   - Identify your service offering?
   - Clarify what needs to be done?
   - Justify why your service is required?
   - Show consideration for the impact on the infrastructure?
   - Explain the cause and effect of the service?

2. **What is your policy/position/philosophy?**

   Can you:
   - Identify your corporate and social responsibility?
   - Explain your fundamental principles?
   - Describe your ethical and moral obligations?
   - Demonstrate your purpose?

3. **What are your returns on investment?**

   Can you:
   - Show your service is financially viable?
   - Substantiate effective use of investment and resources?
   - Demonstrate value for money?
   - Ensure your service is sustainable and show a clear structure for evaluation?

What is a return on investment?

A return on investment is one way of considering profits in relation to capital invested. To ensure investment in school nursing services, commissioners will firstly make a quick assessment of investment performance and secondly compare similar investments over the same time period. A return on investment should be calculated using data to evidence three elements:

- The benefits
- The costs
- The dividends

There are two ways a return on investment can be expressed: in financial terms (which is frequently associated with private industry) or by showing quality measurements (which are often more suitable in healthcare provision).

How do I calculate 'financial' returns on investment?

Whilst it is often difficult to quantify financial returns on investment, there are a range of tariffs and calculations that can be used for guidance.

- Benefits – Costs = Dividends
- (% Figure) Benefits – (Costs × 100)/Costs
- ↓ Tariff payments outweigh the costs of providing the service
- Return on investment calculator
- For further information see: http://www.institute.nhs.uk/

How do I calculate 'quality' returns on investment?

In healthcare provision, commissioners will consider quality returns on investment. This means calculations that can show improvements in care and measurable outcomes.

These improvements may include:

- Reduction in non-attendees
- Reducing illness through prevention
- Lower hospital stay
- Less intensive treatment
- Improving patient experience
- Improved efficiency and effectiveness
- Increased productivity
- Positive staff morale

Many quality indicators are difficult to present, unlike regular financial calculations. However, by using a simple style of approach like the cause and effect relationship (Figure 7.2), quality returns on investments can be demonstrated.

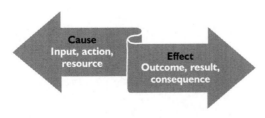

Figure 7.2 Cause and effect (Watson, 2004).

There are a number of studies which help to demonstrate the effectiveness of prevention work which are contained within the HCP document and expressed in financial gains (DH/DCSF, 2009, p. 12):

> ... by investing money now to save greater costs to society in the long term. For example, one American study found that family therapy for young offenders costs an average of $2,380 per participant but saved taxpayers and victims of crime an estimated $52,156 per participant in the longer term (Drake *et al.*, 2009)

How to develop a business case

There are three phases to consider when developing a business case:

Phase 1

Establish a case for change and justify the need.
- Identify a gap in service provision.
- Show the worth of an existing service.
- Justify why the service is needed.
- Provide the evidence.

Phase 2

Evidence a preferred option and describe the new or existing service.
- Overview of service.
- Resources required.
- Evaluation/evidence of success.
- Expected outcomes.

Phase 3

Sell the preferred option using a benefits criteria approach.
- Returns on investment.
- Efficiency, effectiveness and productivity.
- Policy directives and strategy context.
- Sustainability/monitoring.

Once you have collated all your information and data to meet the requirements of all three phases, this can next be presented as a formal business plan.

How to write a business plan using a basic template

See Table 7.6.

Table 7.6 How to write a business plan using a basic template.

Executive summary	■ A summary of the full report ■ Main points of business case ■ Purpose, key messages and recommendations ■ Key objectives for investment
Justification	■ Policy drivers ■ Organisation strategy ■ Research ■ Evidence of need ■ Describe the problem/issues ■ Before picture/benchmark for evaluation
Overview	■ Describe your service ■ Aims and objectives ■ Evaluation process ■ Performance measures
Findings	■ Evaluation ■ Measurements of change/achievements ■ Policy indicators (*equity, efficiency, effectiveness*) ■ Outputs (*evidence, interventions, productivity, resources*) ■ Outcomes (*achieving policy, results, difference/effect*)
Benefits criteria	■ Summarise evaluation ■ Return on investment/value for money ■ Evidence of benefits (patients/clients and staff) ■ Policy indicators (*equity, efficiency, saves money*) ■ Identify obstacles with solutions ■ Gaps and risks analysis ■ Implementation costing
Conclusion	■ Revisit the aims and objectives of the service ■ Summarise the main findings ■ Reinforce the benefits ■ Revisit policy

Improving the efficiency of teams: the Lancaster Model

It is crucial at a time of economic restraint with consequent limited resources that planners of care utilise the skills and knowledge of teams to effectively meet the needs of children and young people. The management and assessment of knowledge and skills is discussed in Chapter 2 with regard to performance management, and the Lancaster Model builds on this by providing a structured model to map these skills and knowledge to local need.

'**The Lancaster Model**' has been rigorously evaluated and is a proven process for securing better outcomes for children, young people and their families (SAPHNA, 2012).

What is the Lancaster Model?

The Lancaster Model has been developed to support school nursing practice, interventions and services through a process of redesign. The main drivers for the development have been the increasing public health challenges facing children, young people and their families and enabling the delivery of the HCP (DH/DCSF 2009) and the School Nurse Development Programme (DH, 2012). The Lancaster Model has been proven to maximise the contribution of school nursing teams without huge financial investment. There are two distinct elements that shape the model. First there is an efficient process that incorporates health and development reviews for children (aged 4–5 years) and young people (aged 10–11 years). This systematic needs assessment approach identifies earlier needs, resources and priorities at individual, neighbourhood and community levels. Second, there is a structured skills analysis strategy which ensures the skills, competencies, experiences, qualifications and training of each individual member of the team are recognised and utilised effectively. The cyclical nature of the model collates ongoing data relating to practice activity and the changing needs of specific users, ensuring that continued service changes and developments are monitored, evaluated and measured against expected outcomes.

The specific aims of the Lancaster Model are to ensure:

1. Effective delivery of the New School Nurse Development Programme (DH, 2012).
2. Delivery of the Healthy Child Programme.
3. Improved team leadership and delegation.
4. More effective targeting of resources to increase earlier interventions.
5. Improved prevention of ill health rather than treating established disease.

In addition to the specific aims, the model also reflects and supports the delivery of a wide range of other changing government policy and strategic indicators (Table 7.7).

How does the Lancaster Model work?

The Lancaster Model is a simple, structured, step-by-step solution to support the delivery of the School Nurse Development Model. There are five easy steps to follow (Figure 7.3):

Table 7.7 Changing government policy.

Policy	Reflected strategic indicator
DH (2010) *Equity & Excellence: Liberating the NHS*. DH, London.	Redesign services to achieve improved quality and efficiency
DH (2010) *Healthy Lives, Healthy People* (Public Health White Paper). DH, London.	Tackle emerging public health challenges by addressing the root causes
Munro, E. (2011) *The Munro Review of Child Protection. Final report. A Child-centred System*. Department of Education, London.	Change reactive services to preventative services
Sir Ian Kennedy (2010) *The Kennedy Review: Getting it Right for Children and Young People* Central Office of Information (COI), London.	Actively engage children, young people and their families in their healthcare
Sustainable Development Unit (2010) *Commissioning for Sustainable Development* NHS Sustainable Development Unit, Cambridge.	Deliver healthcare at the right time, in the right place to the right person
Department of Health (2009) *Achieving Better Outcomes: Commissioning in Children's Services*. DH, London.	Improve outcomes in the most efficient, effective sustainable way
Department of Health (2009) *Transforming Community Services: Enabling New Patterns of Working*. DH, London.	Effectively target resources to need
Department of Health (2010) *Quality, Innovation, Productivity and Prevention – QIPP*. DH, London.	Challenge the way practice is delivered

1. A scoping exercise
2. A sustainable health needs assessment process
3. A skills analysis strategy
4. A workforce redesign template
5. A training support package

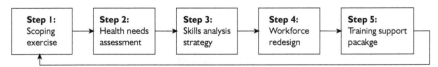

Figure 7.3

Step 1: Scoping exercise

A scoping exercise will establish the interventions and practices that are currently being delivered by the school nursing team. This will provide a benchmark and a point of reference to assess the required future developments and innovations.

Outcomes:

- An up-to-date audit of current service provision
- A review of protocols, processes and service delivery pathways
- An assessment of team compositions and staffing levels
- A mapping of workload allocation
- Identification of any key issues

Step 2: Health needs assessment

The sustainable health needs assessment process provides a cyclical approach of staged contacts to evidence the needs of children, young people and their families. These staged contacts have been designed to incorporate the health and development reviews at school entry (children aged 4–5 years) and at Year 6 (young people aged 10–11 years), as recommended in the Healthy Child Programme.

Outcomes:

- A structured approach to collecting data as part of everyday practice
- A continuum of local user information to influence the commissioning of services
- A universal staged contact at school entry and Year 6
- Health and development reviews to detect individuals with specific needs and risk factors
- A vehicle to enable the delivery of the Healthy Child Programme

Step 3: Skills analysis strategy

The skills analysis strategy will support the redesign of team roles and responsibilities, boundaries of practice and service delivery. This process will establish and recognise the training, knowledge and expertise of each team member regardless of their banding level.

Outcomes:

- A process to distinguish the strengths of existing team members
- Methodology to incorporate existing roles and responsibilities into integrated teams
- Data to evidence boundaries of practice and role overlap
- A strategy to promote team working and collaboration
- Identification of any educational gaps and training needs

Step 4: Workforce redesign

The workforce redesign step will focus on the re-allocation of caseloads, directed by the skills analysis strategy and the evidence derived from the implementation of the Health Needs Assessment Model. This will guide and support delegation of practice and utilise the expertise of all team members.

Outcomes:

- The allocation of caseloads based on need not numbers
- The evidence to ensure services are delivered by competent staff
- A workforce of individuals working within their band and level of capability
- A team with the capacity to lead proactive, innovative public health practice
- A process to support utilising staff from the wider team and other organisations
- The evidence to move and circulate staff to different localities on a yearly cycle

Step 5: A training support programme

A range of training sessions for staff and managers will help to support the implementation of the Lancaster Model. These sessions will also cover leadership, accountability and responsibility, government directives, commissioning and resilience training.

Outcomes:

- A competent workforce to embed the Lancaster Model into practice
- Enhanced knowledge and understanding to support user involvement
- Visionary individuals able to drive policy forward
- Increased motivation and acceptance for transition and change

How can the model improve the effectiveness and efficiency of a team?

The scoping exercise (**Step 1**) uncovers existing practices and interventions by benchmarking current service provision against government directives. At this point unbefitting service provision can be identified and reallocated to the appropriate service provider. Implementation of the needs assessment (**Step 2**) enables school nursing practice to become evidence-based and dependent on the needs of individuals and communities. The skills analysis strategy (**Step 3**) can then be matched to the evidence derived from the needs assessment, to ensure individual team members are working within their competency range and are utilising their knowledge, skills and expertise. While the workforce redesign (**Step 4**) develops, caseload allocation and redirection of resources become structured and needs-led. Each individual team member knows their role and responsibilities and understands why they are delivering specific interventions. The overall result is an increase in team effectiveness and efficiency due to a focused shared vision, improved corporate team working and heightened job satisfaction. The training support programme (**Step 5**), will support and sustain these changes and further developments in the future.

How can the model increase team productivity with current staffing levels and no extra resources?

An increase in team effectiveness and efficiency will automatically result in an increase in team productivity. The word 'productivity' means the ratio of what is produced versus what is required to produce it; this will be shown by the delivery of more interventions and practices by the same existing school nurse team members with no extra resources. This is due to individuals working smarter, not harder, by delivering interventions and services which are focused on evidence and within their range of capability. Ultimately appropriate service provision will be delivered quicker without sacrificing quality. The Lancaster Model is one vehicle that enables the delivery of the School Nurse Development Model, by providing the structures, frameworks and approaches to guide, support and evidence practice, interventions and services through the process of redesign.

How it may map to the school nurse development plan is contained in Box 7.2.

For more information, including a full evaluation of the Lancaster Model, visit http://www.thelancastermodel.co.uk/.

Conclusion

In conclusion, the discipline of school nursing is in an influential position to provide commissioners with information and data with regard to the health and wellbeing of children, young people and their families. The key to successful ongoing investment is ensuring that the content, validity, relevance and delivery of this information and data, supports and influences the commissioning cycle. An increased understanding and acceptance of the process of commissioning will help individual team members to positively support data collection and accept the overall reasons for evidencing need and validating their practice. A formal presentation of this information in the structured format of a business plan will support and assist local commissioners in their decision making.

At last the valuable contribution that a school nursing service has to offer and its unique contribution to improving the health and wellbeing of school aged children and young people has been recognised. The new School Nurse Development

Box 7.2 How the Lancaster Model may link to the School Nurse Development Model

The Lancaster Model

The offer:

- **Your community** (Step 1): The scoping exercise will help to identify who provides the current range of health services available in your community.
- **Universal services** (Step 2): The needs assessment will enable the delivery of the Healthy Child Programme and ensure a healthy start for every child.
- **Universal plus** (Step 3): The skills analysis strategy will support a swift response with specific expert help from members of the team.
- **Universal partnership plus** (Step 4): The workforce redesign will enable ongoing support in partnership from the wider multi-agency teams.
- (Step 5): The training support programme will help and sustain the process throughout.

Model provides direction and development opportunities for existing school nursing teams and a national vision for future investment. Optimism, confidence and a solution-focused approach from all school nursing team members will help to ensure the school nurses are the principle providers of this new way of working. The implementation of models and frameworks such as the Lancaster Model will help to support and help existing teams to start to change the way they work and evidence their unique contribution and value.

References

CNO Chief Nursing Officer Bulletin (2011) *School Nursing Development Programme: the modules.* Available at http://cno.dh.gov.uk/2011/11/24/school-nursing-development-programme-the-modules/ (accessed 21 January 2012).

Department of Health [DH] (2009a) *Transforming Community Services: Enabling New Patterns of Working.* DH, London.

Department of Health (2009b) *Achieving Better Outcomes: Commissioning in Children's Services.* DH, London.

Department of Health (2010) *Action on Health Visiting Programme: Getting it Right for Children and Families.* DH, London.

Department of Health (2012) *Getting it Right for Children, Young People and Their Fami-*

lies. *Maximising the Contribution of the School Nursing Team. Vision and Call to Action*. DH, London.

Department of Health/Department for Children, Schools and Families (2009) *Healthy Child Programme: From 5–19 Years Old*. Department of Health Publications, London.

Drake, K., Aos, S. and Miller, M. G. (2009) Evidence based public health policy options to reduce crime and criminal justice costs. *Victims and Offenders*, 4, 170–96.

New Economics Foundation [NEF] (2009) *A Guide to Commissioning Children's Services for Better Outcomes: Backing the Future – Practical Guide 3*. NEF, London.

Nursing and Midwifery Council (2004) *Standards of Proficiency for Specialist Community Public Health Nurses*. NMC, London.

School and Public Health Nurses Association [SAPHNA] (2012) *The Lancaster Model*. Available at http://www.saphna-professionals.org/node/571 (accessed 20 January 2012).

Watson, G. (2004) The legacy of Ishikawa. *Quality Progress*, **37**(4), 54–7.

Index